S271/14.10.11

Body Work in
and Social Car

Sociology of Health and Illness Monograph Series

Edited by Hannah Bradby
Department of Sociology
University of Warwick
Coventry
CV4 7AL
UK

Current titles

Body Work in Health and Social Care: Critical Themes, New Agendas (2011)
edited by *Julia Twigg, Carol Wolkowitz, Rachel Lara Cohen and Sarah Nettleton*

Technogenarians: Studying Health and Illness Through an Ageing, Science, and Technology Lens (2010)
edited by *Kelly Joyce and Meika Loe*

Communication in Healthcare Settings: Policy, Participation and New Technologies (2009)
edited by *Alison Pilnick, Jon Hindmarsh and Virginia Teas Gill*

Pharmaceuticals and Society: Critical Discourses and Debates (2009)
edited by *Simon J. Williams, Jonathan Gabe and Peter Davis*

Ethnicity, Health and Health Care: Understanding Diversity, Tackling Disadvantage (2008)
edited by *Waqar I. U. Ahmad and Hannah Bradby*

The View From Here: Bioethics and the Social Sciences (2007)
edited by *Raymond de Vries, Leigh Turner, Kristina Orfali and Charles Bosk*

The Social Organisation of Healthcare Work (2006)
edited by *Davina Allen and Alison Pilnick*

Social Movements in Health (2005)
edited by *Phil Brown and Stephen Zavestoski*

Health and the Media (2004)
edited by *Clive Seale*

Partners in Health, Partners in Crime: Exploring the boundaries of criminology and sociology of health and illness (2003)
edited by *Stefan Timmermans and Jonathan Gabe*

Rationing: Constructed Realities and Professional Practices (2002)
edited by *David Hughes and Donald Light*

Rethinking the Sociology of Mental Health (2000)
edited by *Joan Busfield*

Sociological Perspectives on the New Genetics (1999)
edited by *Peter Conrad and Jonathan Gabe*

The Sociology of Health Inequalities (1998)
edited by *Mel Bartley, David Blane and George Davey Smith*

The Sociology of Medical Science (1997)
edited by *Mary Ann Elston*

Health and the Sociology of Emotion (1996)
edited by *Veronica James and Jonathan Gabe*

Medicine, Health and Risk (1995)
edited by *Jonathan Gabe*

Body Work in Health and Social Care
Critical Themes, New Agendas

Edited by

Julia Twigg, Carol Wolkowitz, Rachel Lara Cohen and Sarah Nettleton

WILEY-BLACKWELL

A John Wiley & Sons, Ltd., Publication

This edition first published 2011
Originally published as Volume 33, Issue 2 of *Sociology of Health & Illness*
Chapters © 2011 The Authors
Book compilation © 2011 Foundation for the Sociology of Health & Illness / Blackwell Publishing Ltd

Blackwell Publishing was acquired by John Wiley & Sons in February 2007. Blackwell's publishing program has been merged with Wiley's global Scientific, Technical, and Medical business to form Wiley-Blackwell.

Registered Office
John Wiley & Sons Ltd, The Atrium, Southern Gate, Chichester, West Sussex, PO19 8SQ, United Kingdom

Editorial Offices
350 Main Street, Malden, MA 02148-5020, USA
9600 Garsington Road, Oxford, OX4 2DQ, UK
The Atrium, Southern Gate, Chichester, West Sussex, PO19 8SQ, UK

For details of our global editorial offices, for customer services, and for information about how to apply for permission to reuse the copyright material in this book please see our website at www.wiley.com/wiley-blackwell.

The right of Julia Twigg, Carol Wolkowitz, Rachel Lara Cohen and Sarah Nettleton to be identified as the authors of the editorial material in this work has been asserted in accordance with the UK Copyright, Designs and Patents Act 1988.

Wiley also publishes its books in a variety of electronic formats. Some content that appears in print may not be available in electronic books.

Designations used by companies to distinguish their products are often claimed as trademarks. All brand names and product names used in this book are trade names, service marks, trademarks or registered trademarks of their respective owners. The publisher is not associated with any product or vendor mentioned in this book. This publication is designed to provide accurate and authoritative information in regard to the subject matter covered. It is sold on the understanding that the publisher is not engaged in rendering professional services. If professional advice or other expert assistance is required, the services of a competent professional should be sought.

Library of Congress Cataloging-in-Publication Data

Body work in health and social care : critical themes, new agendas / edited by Julia Twigg... [et al.].
    p. cm. – (Sociology of health and illness monographs ; 10)
    Includes bibliographical references and index.
    ISBN 978-1-4443-4987-0 (pbk.)
    1. Human body–Social aspects.   2. Social medicine.   I. Twigg, Julia.
    HM636.B67 2011
    306.4'61–dc22
                            2011013768

A catalogue record for this book is available from the British Library.

This book is published in the following electronic formats: ePDFs (9781444345834); Wiley Online Library (9781444345865); ePub (9781444345841); Kindle (9781444345858).

Set in 9.5/11.5 pt Times NR Monotype by Toppan Best-set Premedia Limited
Printed in Malaysia by Ho Printing (M) Sdn Bhd

01   2011

Contents

Notes on Contributors

Andy Alaszewski is an Emeritus Professor of the University of Kent, UK. His textbook on *Using Diaries for Social Research* was published by Sage in 2006, and he is editor of the international journal, *Health, Risk and Society*.

Joanna Bornat is Emeritus Professor of Oral History at the Open University, UK. She has a long-standing interest in remembering in late life and continues to research and publish on these topics.

Patrick Brown is an Assistant Professor in the Department of Sociology and Anthropology at the University of Amsterdam. He has published several papers on trust in relation to health policy and is currently writing a book on trust relations within mental health services.

Thea Cacchioni is the Ruth Wynn Woodward Chair in Women's Studies at the University of Victoria, Canada. She has published on women and the medicalisation of sex and testified at an FDA hearing against the approval of a drug proposed to treat low sexual desire in women.

Rachel Lara Cohen is Lecturer at the University of Surrey, UK, and a specialist in sociology of work and employment. She has published articles on the working lives and employment relations of hairstylists. She is currently researching the daily lives of car mechanics and accountants.

Isabel Dyck is Professor of Geography, Queen Mary University of London. She is currently working on a variety of issues related to migration and health, with a particular focus on the home.

Kim England is Professor of Geography at the University of Washington. She is an urban social and feminist geographer who focuses on care work, critical social policy analysis, economic restructuring, and inequalities in North America.

Nicola Gale is a Research Fellow in Medical Sociology at the University of Birmingham, UK. Her main research interests are health beliefs and practices, complementary and alternative medicine, and qualitative methodology in applied health research.

Anna Harris is a postdoctoral researcher at Maastricht University in the Netherlands. She conducted her research on overseas doctors while at the University of Melbourne, Australia, and is currently working on a project concerning genetics and the internet.

Leroi Henry is Senior Research Fellow at The Working Lives Research Institute at London Metropolitan University. His research interests include discrimination in the workplace and the role of social dialogue in restructuring in the public sector.

Elodie Marandet is a PhD student with the Centre for Human Geography at Brunel University, UK. She also worked there as a researcher on a variety of research projects dealing with issues of gender, parenthood and education.

Per Måseide is Professor of Sociology at the University of Nordland, Norway. He has done research on the social organization of medical work, collaborative medical problem solving in hospitals, inter-professional team talk in hospital settings, conceptions of the body in medical work, and the impaired body and use of assistive devices.

Elodie Marandet is a PhD student with the Centre for Human Geography at Brunel University, UK. She also worked there as a researcher on a variety of research projects dealing with issues of gender, parenthood and education.

Sarah Nettleton is Reader in Sociology in the Department of Sociology, University of York, UK. She published *The Sociology of Health and Illness*, Polity Press, 2nd edition.

Mr Andy Nordin is a subspecialist gynaecological oncologist in the East Kent Gynaecological Oncology Centre in Margate, and is an Honorary Senior Lecturer at University College London. He is the National Clinical Advisor to the Department of Health's Cancer Action Team and the NHS Cancer Improvement programme.

Parvati Raghuram is Reader in Human Geography at the Open University. She has written widely on gender, migration and development and is currently theorising migration through a postcolonial lens.

Sadaf Rizvi is a Research Officer at the Institute of Education, University of London, UK. She is a social anthropologist with special interest in anthropology of education and childhood ethnography, and is currently working on learning and life chances in cities.

Chris Shilling is Professor of Sociology and Director of Graduate Studies in SSPSSR at the University of Kent, UK. His books include *Changing Bodies*, Sage, 2008, *The Body in Culture, Technology & Society*, Sage, 2005, and *The Body and Social Theory*, Third Edition, Sage, 2012. He edits The Sociological Review Monograph Series.

Trish Swift was the clinical trials specialist nurse for the East Kent Gynaecological Oncology Centre, based in Margate. She has a research interest in quality of life assessment and was an active member of the EORTC Quality of Life Group until her recent retirement.

Jen Tarr is a Lecturer in Research Methodology at the London School of Economics and Political Science. Her research interests are in the area of qualitative methods, visual and sensory methodologies and somatic practices, including dance.

Julia Twigg is Professor of Social Policy and Sociology at the University of Kent, UK. She published *The Body in Health and Social Care*, Palgrave, 2006, and is currently working on the embodiment of age, in particular clothing and dress.

Emma Wainwright is a Lecturer in the Centre for Human Geography, School of Health Sciences and Social Care at Brunel University, UK. She has led a number of research projects exploring the social geographies of training/education among parents (mothers) and 'non traditional' students.

Carol Wolkowitz is a Reader in the Department of Sociology at the University of Warwick, UK. Her book *Bodies at Work* was published in 2006. She is now researching the development of the 'body work economy' in south Florida.

1

Conceptualising body work in health and social care
Julia Twigg, Carol Wolkowitz, Rachel Lara Cohen and Sarah Nettleton

Introduction

Body work is work that focuses directly on the bodies of others: assessing, diagnosing, handling, treating, manipulating, and monitoring bodies, that thus become the object of the worker's labour. It is a component part of a wide range of occupations. It is a central part of healthcare, through the work of doctors, nurses, dentists, hygienists, paramedics and physiotherapists. It is a fundamental part of social care, particularly for older people in the form of personal care and the work of care assistants (Twigg 2000a). Body work is also a central theme in alternative medicine (Sointu 2006). It is at the heart of the body pleasing, body pampering trades such as hairdressing, beauty work, massage, and tattooing (Black 2004, Sweetman 1999), and it extends to other, more stigmatised occupations, such as sex workers (Sanders 2004, Brents *et al.* 2010) and undertakers (Howarth 1996). The contexts within which these practitioners operate, the knowledge systems they draw on, and the status hierarchies in which they are embedded, vary greatly; however, as we have argued elsewhere (Twigg 2000b, 2006, Wolkowitz 2002, 2006), there are certain commonalities that can be traced across these contexts that make the concept of body work sociologically useful.

This book explores the relevance of the concept of body work for the field of health and social care. The Call for Abstracts followed from a research seminar series organised by the authors in 2007–9 entitled 'Body Work: Critical Issues, Future Agendas' funded by the UK Economic and Social Research Council. The seminars were not confined to the field of health and social care, but brought together social scientists interested in exploring the social relations of body work across a range of occupations that focus on the human body, many of which are far from the conventional areas of health or social care. The series demonstrated how a concept of body work is useful for exploring commonalities and differences in workers' dilemmas and strategies in what are otherwise widely disparate occupations, in ways that highlight, rather than ignore, the particularities of their work. The concept also provided a vehicle for the collaboration of researchers associated with different specialisms, not only those concerned with health and social care, but also scholars of work and employment, gender, ethnicity and migration, and social policy and sociology. The crossovers and commonalities between these fields were among the most fruitful aspects of the seminars. It is very much in the spirit of these wider collaborations that we approach this

Body Work in Health and Social Care, First Edition. Edited by Julia Twigg, Carol Wolkowitz, Rachel Lara Cohen and Sarah Nettleton.
Chapters © 2011 The Authors. Book compilation © 2011 Foundation for the Sociology of Health & Illness / Blackwell Publishing Ltd. Published 2011 by Blackwell Publishing Ltd.

book on body work in health and social care. Indeed, one of the gains of the concept for health and social care is its capacity to link these subjects with wider social structures and discourses.

This introduction to the book seeks to elaborate the concept of body work and to specify some of the gains from adopting it as a focus in health and social care. We begin by highlighting the boundaries and intersections between our conceptualisation of body work and that of parallel and different usages, particularly in relation to emotion, work and the body. We argue that one of the benefits of our definition is to foreground the constraints care of the body must deal with, especially as regards the use of time and space. We suggest that by acknowledging the particular character of body work, we are better able to understand the micro-political relations between practitioners and patients and clients, how difficult these are to alter, and how these are shaped by the wider social and economic context. We are arguing, therefore, that the concept not only makes visible aspects of health and social care too often neglected, but also highlights critical dimensions on which comparative research is needed.

Body work, as we have noted, involves direct, hands-on activities, handling, assessing and manipulating bodies. It is often ambivalent work that may violate the norms of the management of the body, particularly in terms of touch, smell or sight. It is sometimes a form of dirty work in both the literal and sociological senses (Emerson and Pollner 1976) as workers have to negotiate the boundaries of the body and deal with 'matter out of place' (Douglas 1966). Body work also lies on the borders of the erotic, its interventions paralleling and mimicking those of sexuality; and this further reinforces its ambiguous character. It is gendered work, differentially performed by men and women (Widding Isaksen 2002a). It is practised on both an object and a subject and, as such, involves both a knowledge of the materiality of the body and an awareness of the personhood that is present in that body. It can be linked to pleasure and emotional rapport as well as to abuse and discipline. It is ambivalently positioned in relation to power, caught in dynamics that can tip either way, presenting the worker as either a demeaned body servant or an exerciser of Foucauldian biopower. It can treat the body as a unity, or in terms of discrete body parts, and this has implications for how it is organised and experienced. Whether the work takes place on bodily surfaces, or penetrates the body, whether it involves inflicting pain or producing pleasure, whether it deals with the head or the 'nether regions', or appendages rather than the torso may all have implications for the social relations of body work. Body work therefore invokes ontological questions in terms of how the human body is read or known, and how it may be handled, transformed and understood.

Boundaries and intersections

The relations between the body and work have increasingly been the focus of sociological interest (Wolkowitz 2006, Shilling 2005, Gimlin 2007, McDowell 2009). As a result, the term body work has been used in wide and varying ways. It is helpful therefore to clarify what we are and are not including under the terminology, and how our concept of body work relates to other, parallel, conceptualisations. In order to identify a distinct set of social relations, we define 'body work' relatively narrowly. For us, body work involves work that focuses directly on the bodies of others, who thereby become the object of the worker's labour. For reasons of analytic clarity we omit certain areas. Thus work undertaken by individuals on their own bodies, though interesting and increasingly significant, is not included. We omit debates around the self-disciplining of the body as part of the Foucauldian technologies of the self (Foucault 1997), as a requirement for work (Witz *et al.* 2003) or as a project in High Modernity (Shilling 1993), particularly in relation to norms of appearance and control (Bordo 1993, Gimlin 2002, Davis 1995), though we are, of course, interested in the body work of those who are employed to help others meet those expectations, or whose work practices on their own bodies, as Wainwright's chapter in this book shows, are related to their work on others' bodies. We also lay aside the current focus within public health on the requirement for citizens to promote their own health through regimes of bodily activity and control. Again this represents a form of working on the self, not others' bodies. We also exclude the work-transfer occurring in health systems whereby patients take on technology-related activities on their bodies previously performed by staff.

We are also excluding from our concept 'work' that takes place outside the employment nexus, typically in informal, family-based relationships, such as child care or care for frail or elderly relatives, though such activity frequently involves work on the body. Some theorists of care (Ungerson 1997) have argued for the importance of treating it as a unified sector across the public/private divide. Others (Lee Treweek 1996, Twigg 2000a), however, have argued that the distinctive nature of the social relations in which informal care is embedded, and its uncommodified character, mean that it is better analysed apart. For similar reasons we only include voluntary sector body work if organised in ways that mimic paid work. In practice body work tends to be bifurcated in its provision, located either in the informal, family sector or in paid employment. Body work as part of volunteering is an unstable category: too intimate for passing friendship, lacking either the neutrality of paid work or the intimacy and compulsory quality of family relations.

We also exclude work on fragmented bodies and parts of bodies, such as tissue samples or bodily organs. Our focus is on bodies that are whole, and recognisably so. Because of our interest in intersubjectivity, we concentrate on bodies that are alive and, typically, awake to some degree; but we do not exclude work on the dead body, and would include tasks such as laying out the body on the ward, or the work of undertakers in managing and presenting the deceased. In both cases, though the body is dead, the social person is still present in the corpse.

The boundaries of body work are inevitably fluid, and we may on occasion want to work across these boundaries in order to find out when and why they are established and breached in practice. For instance, Rapp (1999) found that when laboratory technicians examining fetal cells found an adverse result they related the sample back to the woman from whom it was taken. We should also note new technologies that enable body work to be conducted 'at a distance'. Laying out these boundaries is helpful in sharpening our concept and clarifying how it is distinctive.

Our use of body work overlaps with that of other theorists. McDowell (2009) adopts the term body work as a shorthand for all the embodied, interactive work in the consumer service sector that requires co-presence. She includes workers' management of their own bodies and bodily performances, not only their attentions to the bodies of patients, clients and customers. McDowell's use of the term is part of her case for bringing the embodied character of many frontline service sector interactions to the fore, and is thus much to be welcomed. In recognising the importance of embodiment in all consumer services encounters she does not, however, adequately distinguish between cases in which workers' focus on the bodies of the clients/customers is a defining and essential feature of the job and other forms of interactive work where the presence of an embodied worker simply adds extra value, pleasure or authority to the interaction (something that has elsewhere been conceptualised as 'aesthetic labour' (Witz *et al.* 2003)). As it happens, many of McDowell's (2009) case studies are examples of body work in our sense, presumably because they best illustrate the usefulness of looking at the corporeality of interactions in the construction of jobs and occupational identities. However, we think that occupations that require touching the patient or client's body (or at least close proximity or inspection) are characterised by particular challenges and dilemmas and that these are analysed more sharply by confining the term to those situations.

'Body work' also overlaps, empirically and theoretically, with the alternative conceptualisation of 'intimate labour' (Boris and Parreñas 2010), a concept rooted in discussions of the increasing commercialisation of intimacy (Hochschild 2003a, Zelizer 2005). This concept, however, is as much concerned with the transformation of the social experiences of consumers as providers; and this has meant that domestic labour, much of which does not involve intimate touch, is included, as it occurs within the intimacy of the consumer's home. We suggest that our concept of body work has a key advantage over 'intimate labour', in that the focus on intimacy can elide the bodily nature of the work. If working closely with bodies is simply associated with 'intimacy', it becomes essentially an intense form of emotional labour (Hochschild 1983), implying a difference of degree rather than kind. This is not to say that emotional and body work are not closely intertwined, but that the bodily aspects of the work need to be analytically distinguished.

As we have noted, body work inevitably involves an interplay of inter-subjectivities. There has already been much written about emotional labour (Hochschild 1983, Bolton and Boyd 2003, Kang 2003) and this literature needs to be incorporated in the conceptualisation of body work. Although the concept of 'emotional labour' was initially developed within the commercial service sectors, sociologists of health and illness have also recognised and demonstrated that working with, for and on bodies in health and social care settings is emotionally draining, laborious and demanding (James 1989, 1992). 'Emotional labour' maps neatly on to the gendered occupational hierarchies of healthcare, with the privileged, predominantly male professions relegating the emotional work, along with the other 'dirty work', to those lower down the pecking order. There is empirical evidence to support this; though it is important to note that those in the upper echelons of the healthcare division of labour are not immune from emotional 'wear and tear' (Graham 2006, Nettleton et al. 2008). Feelings, both physical and emotional, potentially involve vulnerability, and since the whole edifice of biomedical science, and attendant evidence-based practice, presupposes a form of 'disembedded' expertise (Giddens 1990), the viable scope for emotions becomes awkward, and much emotional work involves the suppression, rather than expression, of emotion. Thus, while emotional sensitivity and expressivity are desired and necessary characteristics of medical work, they must be circumscribed lest they are conceived of as 'unprofessional' and a threat to the abstract system of medicine (Nettleton et al. 2008).

It is important to recognise that not all the emotional aspects of body work are negative. Emotion can also make body work worthwhile, meaningful and rewarding. It is double-edged: a source of satisfaction and frustration. For many, the affective aspects of work constitute an important motivation and are a welcome counter to the encroachments of bureaucratic tasks (Bolton 2005, Cohen 2010). Body workers are likely to experience empathy and sympathy, not least in settings where the women, men, boys and girls with whom, and on whom, they work are facing profound life events or death. But they are also exposed to hurt by those on whom they practice. As we discuss further, below, the power relations are not unilateral and, when dealing with people, practitioners can experience sexism, racism, and other forms of abuse. The emotional component of body work has thus to be managed as part of the job. It also transcends and permeates boundaries between formal paid employment and the lives beyond, for emotions generated through body work are not easily shed or cast off when the worker leaves the workplace, especially when the workplace is a health and social care setting.

Making body work visible

Though the body is central to the activities of health and social care, this fact is often obscured in accounts of the sector. The reasons for this are complex and relate to both the ontological and sociological status of the body and work on it, and to features specific to the construction and analysis of health and social care work. Medicine, for example, is marked by a 'dematerialising tendency' (Dunlop 1986: 664) whereby status is marked by distance from the body, so that when high status professions like doctors do engage in body work they do so in ways whereby the body element is closely framed, with the potentially demeaning aspects of it bracketed off, either symbolically through the use of distancing techniques, like the drama of the ward round or pre-surgical cloaking, or transferred across to lesser status, ancillary, and frequently gendered, occupations like nursing (Twigg 2000a). Similar processes operate within nursing, where status is once again marked by distance from the body. Nursing has often been oddly coy about the reality of frontline bed and body work which has been rarely articulated in nursing texts or discourse (Lawler 1991, 1997). Nurses, as they progress up the occupational hierarchy, move away from the basic – from 'dirty' work on bodies to 'clean' work on machines – and eventually to work, like management or teaching, that involves little or no body work at all. This retreat from body work has been reinforced by the growing division of labour within nursing through the use of skill mix, allied to the long-running desire of nursing to establish its professional status. Social care has similarly avoided thinking of itself in terms of body work. Social care is traditionally constituted in the discourses of social work and managerialism, neither of which emphasise the bodily (Twigg 2006). Social work in particular has traditionally defined its role as 'not the body', handing that territory over to medicine (Diamond 1992). But social care is in fact centrally about body care, which forms the main activity of residential and home care.

The methods used to explore this territory in health and social care research also tend to downplay the bodily. Empirical research is dominated by interviews, in which the experiences of workers and patients are translated into words, with the inevitable bias towards abstraction and bleaching out of the corporeal. There is paucity of observational work. Partly this is because access to the private world of body care is not easy to negotiate: care acts take place in private spaces; and staff act to protect the dignity of patients and, significantly, themselves, for as Lawler (1991) showed in her classic account of nursing, nurses go 'behind the screens' not only to protect the dignity of patients but also of themselves as caring, 'clean' professionals. As Lawton (2003) argues there is a need for novel methodological approaches. Significantly it is ethnographic and observational studies, particularly those like Diamond (1992) and Lee-Treweek (1994, 1996, 1998) based on participant observation, that have cast most light on the embedded and embodied nature of body work. Fields like carework that involve 'unskilled' labour can allow for participant observation by researchers, whereas healthcare interventions, though they take place in more public settings, may not be open to researchers in the same way, and this may obscure our embodied knowledge of them. Harris's chapter in this book is thus particularly welcome for its first-hand reflection on embodied practice by a doctor. The increasingly stringent ethical guidelines that regulate social research particularly in relation to privacy and consent (Boden et al. 2009) may also militate against such techniques.

Time, space and place

The spatial and temporal ordering of body work is central to its provision. Body work requires co-presence. Workers and the bodies they work upon must be in the same place. Moreover, they must be in the same place at the same time. This makes the times and places of body work relatively inflexible. It also has a series of other consequences. First, techno-logical innovations notwithstanding, it is unlikely that body work will ever be comprehen-sively off-shored, that is, exported overseas to lower wage economies. Since the bodies in need of work – patients, clients or customers – remain geographically dispersed, both within and across countries, so does demand for body work. This does not however mean that paid body work is evenly spread geographically. A second consequence is that since the resources required to pay for bodily needs, whether these are for healthcare or personal adornment, are unevenly distributed, so too is paid body work, with a greater concentration of body workers in rich countries and regions. This in turn generates a further consequence in the demand for and immigration of workers, many of whom come from countries with less developed paid body work economies, producing what have become known as 'global care chains' (Hochschild 2003b, Yeates 2004). Within countries, however, the spatial dis-persal can also reflect longer established patterns of living arrangements and employment, with coastal and other retirement areas populated by low-income, frail older people, and with economies of care that draw on unskilled local labour.

In addition to workers' spatial mobility, the global market for body work increasingly depends on the ability of bodies (patients or customers) to travel to sites of regional spe-cialisation. This travel is found in health and social care, for example 'medical tourism' (Connell 2006), but also in other types of body work, for example, 'sex tourism' (O'Connell Davidson 1996) or even the search for obscure and culturally 'authentic' tattoo design (DeMello 2000: 14). 'Tourism' tags notwithstanding, some travel for body work results in permanent relocation, either locally, into long-stay nursing homes or further afield, as in the case of the steady stream of retirees moving to Spain, Florida and other sunbelt regions (Katz 2005, Wolkowitz 2010b). The permanent relocation of people who are particularly needy in terms of their demands for body work reinforces incipient spatial variation in body work demand and its corollary, patterns of global labour migration.

In order to achieve the co-presence necessary for body work in health and social care, workers must make themselves available not just in the right region but in the specific places and at the times that the bodies of patients, clients or service users are ready to be worked on. This may be difficult to manage within capitalist wage-labour relations. Body time fits poorly with 'clock time' (Simmonds 2002). Whereas clock time, the commodity against which capitalist wage-labour is reckoned (Adam 1993), is abstract, accountable and exchangeable, bodily rhythms are individual and variable, the times and duration of bodily need unpredictable and expansive, as Davies (1994) showed in her account of what she terms the 'process time' of care. The dependence of the body work labour process on bodily needs makes it difficult to rationalise or speed up, as Cohen argues in this book. Since many bodily needs are difficult to constrain to 'working hours', body work is potentially 24 hours a day 365 days a year, requiring flexible bodies and flexible workers (Martin 1994). Moreover, the unpredictable nature of body work means that demand spikes are inevitable. When these occur, unless staffing levels are 'unprofitably' high, a decreasing likelihood given the dominance of the profit-motive in the social organisation of body work, some demand is likely to go unmet; patients, clients or service users left waiting, as Diamond's (1992) account of for-profit care homes showed.

The site where body work takes place is also significant. Body work can take place both within and outside designated workplaces, with the same task taking on very different features depending on where it occurs. For example, a care assistant who washes the body of an older person in a residential care home will be subject to the institution's schedule, conscious of the other bodies awaiting attention and perhaps subject to direct surveillance by a manager or to intervening demands from other residents (Diamond 1992, Lopez 2006). The same tasks may be performed in a private home and may be similarly rushed, with the timetable determined by the minutes allotted to each visit, but the spaces and times of work are here produced and managed not only by an external manager but in direct relationship with the person being washed, and the family or friends who form their social network (as England and Dyck explore in this book). Body work that takes place in domestic spaces can thus both extend commodification, whilst simultaneously removing waged labour from direct managerial control and embedding it within extra-economic social spatial and temporal relationships.

Much of the meaning of these relationships derives from the fact that these activities take place in a distinctive and special space, that of home (Rubenstein 1989, Sixsmith 1990, Allen and Crow 1987, Gurney and Means 1993). The coming of care, particularly intimate body care, into this ordered space disrupts its meanings, challenges its privacies, and redistributes its spaces, as Twigg (1999) and Angus and colleagues (2005) showed in their analyses of home care. There is interplay between the body and its structured privacy and that of the spatial ordering of the home. The provision of bodily care also interacts with the temporal ordering of the home, intruding into its structured round of privacy and intimacy, at times presenting disjunctive social experiences in which the body is dressed, undressed, washed and bathed at 'meaningless' times that conflict with normal social ordering, and that impose on it the rationalised clock-based time of bureaucratic provision (Twigg 2000a).

Divisions of labour

Paying attention to the social meanings of body work also helps to explain why the social division of labour in health and social care is so resistant to change. Resonating through the provision of body work are a series of assumptions about gender, class, race and age that shape the pattern of provision and its social evaluation. The mind-body binary is a strongly gendered construction, with the body identified with women and the mind identified men (Grosz 1994). Ungerson (1983) and Widding Isaksen (2002b) argue that women's much greater involvement in bodily care rests on normative associations in relation to gender, bodies, spatial regulations – and dirt. Widding Isaksen (2002a) argues that 'masculine dignity' is much more dependent on fantasies of the body as closed and bounded, and consequently men find care work psychically challenging and fearful. Many of the positive cultural associations of body work, including touch as comforting or healing, are also seen as feminine, drawing on deeply entrenched patterns in relation to motherhood. Body work, as we have noted, also borders on the ambiguous territory of sexuality. Hegemonic masculinity constructs men as potentially sexually predatory (Connell 1995), and this means that limits are often placed on their access to bodies, both female and male; women by contrast are accorded greater freedom, their intervention being interpreted as sexually neutral or safe. As a result, many patients and clients, both male and female, display a preference for receiving care from women. This further underpins the gendered character of body care, with women greatly overrepresented in both paid and unpaid care work; and with further repercussions for the gender segmentation of the labour market as a whole.

The Cartesian division of responsibilities of brain and body is classed and raced, as well as gendered. In Britain, the Victorians gave working-class women responsibility for the sexualised and cloacal 'nether regions' of the body, allowing the middle-class lady to maintain the purity essential to her role as society's heart. In relation to nursing in the 19th century, however, as Bashford (1998) shows, it was chaste, young, middle-class women who were entrusted as part of the sanitary enterprise with the care of bodies. Since then the growing division of labour in healthcare and the changing social base of nursing have shifted the body work of healthcare over to less elite workers. Nowadays, responsibility for caring for the body, including both children and the elderly, is highly dependent on classed and racialised groups (Neysmith and Aronson 1997, Anderson 2000); and this reinforces the stigma that serving the body carries.

We also need to note the relevance of the social meanings attached to different bodies. Bodily differences may sometimes have a physical dimension, such as the frailty of older bodies. At other times differences are not due to physical power but nonetheless take a bodily form, such as racialised or class markers of social hierarchy. These differences may be rendered more salient, for both worker and recipient, by the close bodily intimacy of body work. Moreover, some bodies may be seen as particularly polluting. For instance, Widding Isaksen, whose account concentrates on elder care, drawing on Kubie and Lawler (1991), argues that the ageing body is seen to carry a 'piling up of undischarged remnants of a lifetime of eating and drinking...' and thus perceived as particularly dirty, 'open, unlimited and unattractive' (Widding Isaksen 2002b: 802, 792). Contrasts can be drawn here between the stigmatised bodies of many who receive health and social care and the more privileged bodies of those in receipt of the body pampering, body enhancing treatment of the beauty, wellbeing and sex work industries (Black 2004, Sanders 2004), though these groups of recipients are themselves very varied. The status of the bodies treated has important consequences for the organisation of body work and the power dynamics of body care.

The power relations of body work

Focusing on the body work of health and social care highlights the corporeality of power relations between practitioners and patients or clients and the corporeal inter-dependence that characterises their interactions. Generally speaking, the power relations of healthcare tend to advantage the practitioner or worker over and above the immediate recipient of his or her attentions (Wolkowitz 2002). This is partly because the practitioner's social class – though also often their gender and age status – is frequently superior to that of the patient. This is especially so in the case of doctors and dentists, but sometimes also in nursing (Chambliss 1996, Abel and Nelson 1990). Practitioners' relative power also rests on forms of expertise and organisational authority that specify how the body is to be treated (Wolkowitz 2011). Studying the body work of healthcare thus shifts attention to the immediate micropolitics of care, including the ways the institutional power of healthcare practitioners is embodied through interaction with patients (and occasionally undermined). For instance, the physical postures and positioning of the practitioner and client or patient necessitated by any particular treatment will affect their interaction. Can they look each other in the eye? Will one be standing and the other lying down? Is one dressed for public interactions and the other not? The interaction between body worker and recipient may also be influenced by differences in physical strength and ability, especially in those instances where recipients are relatively frail. Even people who are normally hale and hearty may be rendered physically vulnerable through their treatment, at least temporarily.

Body work involves work on both an object body and a subject person, but routinised and standardised health and social care practices construct the recipients of care as tractable and predictable, transforming their bodies into appropriate objects of labour. Looking at health and social care as body work helps to make visible the ways practitioners achieve this, effecting their institutional power within the interaction. The clearest case of this is surgery, where sedation plays the main role in producing a passive 'patient-body', although, as Moreira (2004: 116) suggests, the positioning of the patient starts much earlier, through preoperative procedures during admissions and on the ward. The interpersonal, emotional work undertaken by healthcare practitioners to solicit the willing participation of the patient (see Måseide, and Cacchioni and Wolkowitz, in this book) also frequently has an 'instrumental' character (Theodosius 2008), designed to produce a compliant patient or to distract her from pain. Healthcare practitioners also, wittingly or otherwise, discourage interactions and requests for help from patients through their body language (Halford and Leonard 2003). Practitioners of complementary and alternative medicine (CAM) usually articulate a more equalitarian view of practitioner-patient relations than those in allopathic medicine (Oerton 2004, Sointu 2006), but it is not by chance that their healthcare practices do not generally require the infliction of pain or the immobilisation of the patient, so that the micropolitics of their interactions rarely challenge the equalitarian ethos.

Although the dependence of the practitioner on the compliance of the patient provides many opportunities for patients' resistance, in the context of immediate interactions these are rarely acknowledged, never mind encouraged. Hence one is likely to find that expressions of resistance either burst out in unpredictable ways (racial and other forms of verbal abuse that patients inflict on nurses and other carers (Gunaratnam 2001)); or they take place distant from the immediate encounter, for instance through the organisation of self-help groups or users' support networks. Attempts to empower patients through more patient choice may do little to reduce patients' feelings of vulnerability, since these discourses hardly address the physical vulnerability of patients within body work encounters where they are often naked, prone, weak, subject to the surveillance and control of stronger, clothed staff. The micropolitics of the body work interaction is one reason why the power of patients, even private, fee-paying patients, is limited, as Twigg (2000a) found in her study of the provision of bathing where even wealthy and elite recipients were reduced in power and status by the bodily dynamics of the intervention.

Healthcare practitioners' relative power vis-a-vis patients is especially striking in comparison to the power relations of consumer services in body work. Where customers are seen as entitled to exercise control (or at least the fiction of consumer sovereignty), as in the beauty and body-building industries, workers try to demonstrate that they put the customer and her/his wishes first (Korczynski 2008, Kang 2003, 2010, George 2008, Gimlin 1996, Cohen 2010). Power relations in these interactions may mirror wider status differentials between the working-class hairdresser, manicurist or personal trainer and the middle-class client, but even here power may have to be tangibly acknowledged. For instance, Black suggests that beauticians develop a 'light and compliant touch' (2004: 119) that emphasises the client's relative power within the interaction. However, the fact that aesthetic workers seek to reassure the client, establish trust, through touch and in other ways (Eayrs 1993), suggests that where body work involves nudity or (even temporary) immobility the potential for the worker's exercise of power over the customer is always present. The exercise of physical power is therefore likely to be characteristic of most body work interactions to some degree at least.

The power relations of care work forms an interesting case, since the worker does not usually have the authority of a doctor, nor does the patient typically have the power conferred by consumer ideology. The care worker is usually a woman, sometimes a migrant worker, holding an ill-paid job, with little social status, and moreover one that is often stigmatised because of the dirty work it involves. Even her employer tends to devalue her contribution (Pfefferie and Weinberg 2008). Patients and clients have the power to 'act up', to refuse treatment or care, or to make it difficult for the worker to perform. However, as Lee-Trewick's (1996) study of residential care suggested, care workers have plenty of opportunities to retaliate, including the withdrawal of emotional support. Nonetheless, as England and Dyck in this book suggest, longstanding care relations often mingle respect and concern with physical care, and this gives both worker and client opportunities to influence the other in ways that are not dissimilar to those of other affective relationships.

The links between body work and wider social and economic change

Although focusing on body work draws particular attention to the close bodily proximity of practitioners and patients, it is important to recognise that its performance is inevitably shaped by wider social and economic forces and demographic trends. The question of whether or not a mutually respectful relationship between worker and recipient can be sustained needs to take account of the three-way relation between the worker or practitioner, their employer, and the client or patient (MacDonald and Sirianni 1996). Moreover, the state plays a major role as a fourth party, funding care provided by private businesses or practitioners, even when not providing it directly through public services, as well as through establishing regulatory care standards and specifying staffclient ratios (Himmelweit 2005).

Two wider shifts in the provision of body work services are now widely recognised. First is the substantial increase in the size of the body work labour force in the global North, with the population of most of these countries ageing, and thus requiring more care. Meanwhile the rise in women's paid employment has left a 'care deficit' in the care of young children and the infirm ageing population that is being filled with paid employees (Hochschild 2003b, Folbre and Nelson 2000). Hence healthcare and personal support occupations are among the fastest growing occupations (Bureau of Labor Statistics 2003). Cohen (this book) estimates that at least 10% of the UK labour force is employed in occupations which involve body work, with over half of that figure employed in health and social care. Wolkowitz (2010) estimated that the equivalent figure for the US, even as far back as 2002 was 8%. A labour force of this size is bound to be subject to rationalisation and the development of systems of delivery that abstract from the corporeal relation at its heart.

Secondly, the performance of body work is increasingly dependent on migrant workers or other racialised groups. Immigrant doctors and nurses have played an important role in the provision of healthcare since the inception of the National Health Service in Britain (see Raghuram and colleagues in this book), but in recent years the domestic care deficit has been filled by different groups of 'subordinate-race' women or other migrants in different parts of the globe, with regional differences within countries (Glenn 2001, Foner 1994, Solari 2006, Lan 2006, Parreñas 2006, Guevarra 2006). Body work is therefore embedded in a global division of reproductive labour that, with the partial exception of doctors and dentists, is feminised and racialised.

The performance of body work, however, is linked to, and shaped by, the wider social and economic forces in less obvious ways: body work in health and social care is now deeply integrated into the wider global political economy dominated by forms of capitalist rationality in the management of resources, including labour. As noted above, it has become part of the wider category of services that, because they require co-presence, cannot be offshored on a large scale (Blinder 2006, Gatta *et al.* 2009, McDowell 2009). The financial gains accruing from the provision of high tech expertise to support new body practices such as transplants, assisted reproduction, genomic research, and sex reassignment are legion (Dickenson 2007, Lowe 1995), as is the provision of specialised or high-tech healthcare services for the 'lucrative market' of international patients (Lee and Davis 2004).

Even the more mundane kinds of health and social care have become a source of profit. Public authorities cannot export the processing of bodies overseas to lower wage economies, at least not on a large scale, but they can open up health and social care to private corporations in the expectation that for-profit firms will be better able to organise public services efficiently. However, when health and care are treated just like any other productive services, as is increasingly the case (McDonald and Ruiters 2006, Greer 2008, Player and Lees 2008), the distinctive requirements of body work as a labour process may disappear from the reckoning and the stage will be set for disputes over setting standards of care. The transformation of personal care services for the functionally impaired segment of the ageing population is the best demonstration of this trend. Because much of this care is funded by the state, either directly, through national health services or local authorities, or indirectly, through health and social care programmes for the aged or indigent, such as Medicare or Medicare in the US, the actual provision of care is a potentially profitable business activity (Diamond 1992, Howes 2004, Gatta *et al.* 2009). In the UK, for instance, the proportion of domiciliary care provided by the independent sector, but funded partly by the state, increased from 2% to 70% between 1992 and 2009, and is now worth some £1.5 billion, with some firms responsible for up to 15,000 care recipients (Snell 2009).

The privatisation of residential and domiciliary care services is argued to affect the quality of care along with the relationship between careworker and recipient. Diamond (1992) argues that privatising nursing homes turns care 'into a commodity and the residents into manageable units' (1992: 204). Calculation of 'the bottom line' becomes possible only when 'everyday needs and tending to them' are 'turned into a countable, accountable logic' (1992: 209). However, the same transformation also takes place when care provided directly by public bodies, or funded by them, has to conform to strict budgeting criteria. Campbell's (2008) discussion of a Canadian ethnography of domiciliary care suggests that standardised timings inevitably ignore the diverse circumstances in which a bath or other care work is actually done. Building on the work of Dorothy Smith (1988), Campbell argues that embodied clients come to exist only on paper, as the 'textualised' creations of bureaucratised systems of service delivery. According to Lopez (2006), time-pressed workers have less latitude to adapt their routines to patients' wishes, and will need instead to push them through their daily routines. Hence, improvements in the treatment of care home residents depend much more on dealing with structured constraints, especially understaffing, than on changing organisational cultures.

In other cases, privatisation takes the form of turning the client or their relatives into employers; this may enable some care users to feel more empowered, but has mixed or detrimental consequences for workers (Benjamin and Matthias 2004). Several commentators argue that funding arrangements to empower patients have followed the demands of campaigns by disabled younger men and reinforce an ideology of individual independence that is less relevant to other groups of people needing personal assistance (Ungerson 1993, Watson *et al.* 2004). There may also be a more fundamental problem with measures that maintain the disabled person's sense of personal independence at the cost of the selfeffacement, or relative disempowerment, of the worker's status (Ungerson 1999, Rivas 2003). As Razavi (2007) suggests, the links between service quality and working conditions needs to be better publicised. Following from this, campaigns to empower patients and clients may be most effective when practitioners and patients (or their relatives) form coalitions that defend workers' rights, pay and conditions (Boris and Klein 2006, Lopez 2006).

Conclusion

In this introductory chapter we have tried to identify some of the characteristics of body work, its links with existing areas of research interest, and the new insights it can promote. Conceptualising body work means paying attention to the proximate character of frontline work in health and social care, including the implications of the physicality of the body and constructions of its meanings for workers in health and social care, the emotional demands such work makes and the ways in which the interactions between clients and patients are experienced through and in the body. We suggest that the concept of body work, with its explicit focus on the interaction of practitioners with patients' and clients' bodies and how these are understood, helps to explain the status hierarchies in health and social care and their intersection with gender, 'race' and ethnicity. Because of its capacity to bridge the gap between large-scale planning and practitioner-patient interactions, the concept of body work is germane to a number of policy issues. Body work needs to be studied within and across healthcare regimes, so that one can trace the tangible effects of changes in the organisation of services, funding, and other 'external' constraints on how body work is structured, measured, monitored and experienced. The concept of body work is especially useful in capturing the variability and timeliness of human needs for care and the costs for patients and workers of failing to allow for this, and therefore the contradictions inherent in the provision of care guided by measures of efficiency and standardised protocols.

In the chapters that follow, a range of scholars explore the significance of body work across a variety of settings and professions. Rachel Lara Cohen opens the debate with a wideranging analysis of the labour process of body work, laying out the constraints imposed by the nature of bodies. Contrasting health and care with other service sectors, she highlights the labour intensity of body work, showing how it is difficult to concentrate or standardise spatially or temporally because of the unpredictable nature of the body and its needs. She points to the way in which attempts to generate efficiency savings in health and social care are costly for workers and for the bodies that are worked upon.

Kim England and Isabel Dyck deepen the analysis ethnographically with their exploration of the distinctive negotiations that structure the body work of care in the home environment. Drawing on qualitative data from Ontario, Canada, they highlight the negotiated nature of the work, showing how successfully caring for the body in the home environment inevitably involves the formation of both a division of labour *and* strong, co-operative relationships between family caregivers, care workers and care receivers.

Emma Wainwright, Elodie Marandet and Sadaf Rizvi turn the lens of their analysis on to training, providing insights into the ways in which working-class mothers are made into body workers. Drawing on qualitative interviews with mothers training for a range of body work occupations (child care, carework, nursing, massage reflexology, aromatherapy and beauty work) they show that becoming a body worker requires extensive disciplining of one's own body. Perhaps surprisingly, given the gendered nature of body work, this disciplinary process, which they term 'body training', is partly focused on eliminating overt displays of femininity, especially female sexuality.

Continuing the theme of training, Nicola Gale draws on an ethnographic study of trainee practitioners of osteopathy and homeopathy, analysing their experiences of learning their craft and the ways this involves understanding how to communicate and touch the patient's body. In making sense of the activities and practices of these complementary and alternative practitioners, she introduces two novel concepts: 'listening to body talk' and 'body stories'. Listening to body talk encapsulates the contribution of the active patient. Patients here, unlike in the situation analysed by Måseide (this book), do not have to be technically competent but do need a degree of communicative competency to articulate their symptoms. This in turn relates to the 'body stories' whereby the interactional ability of both practitioner and patient give rise to an effective narration of the symptoms and concerns that require attention.

Jennifer Tarr in her chapter focuses upon what she sees as irresolvable tensions between biomedicine and Alexander Technique. She contends that the discursive claims and strategies pursued by practitioners of the Technique hinder any reconciliation or acceptance of their practice by mainstream medicine. In particular, and drawing on ethnographic data, she maintains that proponents and practitioners emphasise that they work upon the 'self' and the conscious body. The integration of the mind and body is crucial; any attempt to alter the physical body alone would be unsuccessful. Thus she concludes that an incompatibility lies in the discursive frameworks which privilege the integration of the mind/self and body over the objective body in contrast to those of the objective body of biomedicine.

Thea Cacchioni and Carol Wolkowitz's chapter turns to medicine and the intimate body work that doctors and physiotherapists may offer women seeking treatment for sexual pain disorders. Their interviews and observations in Vancouver suggest that successful treatment depends on engaging with the cultural meanings of the vagina. The careful negotiation of touch formed part of the treatment, and is not simply a way of negotiating access to the patient's sexual organs. These practitioners' engagement with both bodily and social dimensions of women's perceived sexual difficulties runs counter to the polarisation of physiological and social factors that has characterised debate on the medicalisation of sex.

Patrick Brown, Andy Alaszewski, Trish Swift and Andy Nordin continue the theme of intimacy and touch in their chapter on gynae-oncological encounters. They reflect on the element of trust in the medical encounter, focusing in particular on the embodied quality of interactions on which trust is based. They show how trust is embodied in and through body work, and how seemingly detached forms of body work are connected with the emotion work of care and the craft work of body work as touch.

Drawing on his observational study of respiratory physiological clinics in Norway, Per Måseide again explores the nature of medical examination, though in this case the 'body work' involves no direct hands-on work or touching of the patient's body, as the examination process is mediated by technology used to measure the patient's physiological status. The 'correct' use of the equipment requires effective communication between the doctor and patient, with the former working to ensure compliance on the part of the latter, so that the body work entails the constitution of an active, able and compliant patient. Måseide argues that the examination represents a mutually constitutive process between bodies and bodily modes; their agency and objectification are evident throughout the medical assessment.

Anna Harris shows how looking at doctors' body work sheds light on challenges facing migrant doctors that are often obscured by the more usual concentration on formal qualifications. Her auto-ethnography of her experience as an overseas doctor beginning to practise in the UK concentrates on the 'moment of mismatch' she experienced when working in an unfamiliar environment, one that made conscious the taken-for-granted embodied, tactile learning that medical practice requires.

Parvati Raghuram, Joanna Bornat and Leroi Henry deepen the exploration of the intersections between the bodies of workers and of patient/clients by once again focusing on migrant doctors, this time those caring for frail older people. Drawing on oral history interviews with South Asian geriatricians who worked in the UK, they trace the complex interplay between the stigmatised bodies of older people in the healthcare system and the racialised bodies of the migrant doctors assigned to care for them.

Finally Chris Shilling uses his Afterword to reflect upon the contribution of classical sociological theory to the conceptualisation of the field of body work.

References

Abel, E.K. and Nelson, N.K. (1990) *Circles of Care*. Albany: State University of New York.

Adam, B. (1993) Within and beyond the time economy of employment relations: conceptual issues pertinent to research on time and work, *Social Science Information*, 32, 163–84.

Allan, G. and Crow, G. (eds) (1989) *Home and Family: Creating the Domestic Sphere*. London: Macmillan.

Anderson, B. (2000) *Doing the Dirty Work? The Global Politics of Domestic Labour*. London: Zed Books.

Angus, J.E., Kontos, P., Dyck, I., McKeever, P. and Poland, B. (2005) The physical significance of home: habitus and the experience of receiving long term home care, *Sociology of Health and Illness*, 27, 2, 161–87.

Aronson, J. and Neysmith, S.M. (1996) 'You're not just there to do the work': depersonalizing policies and the exploitation of home care workers' labor, *Gender and Society*, 10, 1, 59–77.

Bashford, A. (2000) *Purity and Pollution: Gender, Embodiment and Victorian Medicine*. Basingstoke: Macmillan.

Benjamin, A.E. and Matthias, R.E. (2004) Work-life differences and outcomes for agency and consumer directed home-care workers, *The Gerontologist*, 44, 4, 479–88.

Blinder, A.S. (2006) Offshoring: the next industrial revolution, *Foreign Affairs*, 85, 2, 113–28.

Black, P. (2004) *The Beauty Industry: Gender, Culture, Pleasure*. London: Routledge.

Boden, R., Epstein, D. and Latimer, J. (2009) Accounting for ethos or programmes for conduct? The brave new world of research ethics committees, *Sociological Review*, 57, 4, 727–49.

Bolton, S.C. (2005) *Emotion Management in the Workplace*. Basingstoke: Palgrave.

Bolton, S.C. and Boyd, C. (2003) Trolley dolly or skilled emotion manager? Moving on from Hochschild's managed heart, *Work, Employment and Society*, 17, 2, 289–308.

Boris, E. and Klein, J. (2006) Organizing home care, *Politics and Society*, 34, 1, 81–108.

Boris, E. and Parreñas, R.C. (2010) *Intimate Labors: Cultures, Technologies and Politics of Care*. Palo Alto, CA: Stanford University Press.

Brents, B.G., Jackson, C.A. and Hausbeck, K, (2010) *The State of Sex: Tourism, Sex, and Sin in the New American Heartland*. New York: Routledge.

Bureau of Labor Statistics (BLS) *Occupational Outlook Handbook 2008–9* http://www.bls.gov/oco/oco2003.htm Accessed on 20/4/09.

Campbell, M. (2008) (Dis)continuity of care. In DeVault, M. (ed.) *People at Work*. NY: New York University Press.

Cant, S. and Sharma, U. (1999) *A New Medical Pluralism? Alternative Medicine, Doctors and Patients and the State*. London: UCL Press.

Chambliss, D. (1996) *Beyond Caring: Hospitals, Nursing and the Social Organisation of Ethics*. Chicago: University of Chicago Press.

Cohen, R.L. (2010) When it pays to be friendly: employment relationships and emotional labour in hairstyling, *Sociological Review*, 58, 197–218.

Connell, J. (2006) Medical tourism: sea, sun, sand and . . . surgery, *Tourism Management*, 27, 1093–100.

Connell, R.W. (1995) *Masculinities*. Cambridge: Polity.

Coward, R. (1989) *The Whole Truth: the Myth of Alternative Medicine*. London: Faber.

Davies, K. (1994) The tensions between process time and clock time in care-work: the example of day nurseries, *Time Society*, 3, 277–303.

Davis, K. (1995) *Reshaping the Female Body: the Dilemma of Cosmetic Surgery*. London: Routledge.

DeMello, M. (2000) *Bodies of Inscription: a Cultural History of the Modern Tattoo Community*. Durham, NC: Duke University Press.

Diamond, T. (1992) *Making Gray Gold: Narratives of Nursing Home Care*. Chicago: University of Chicago Press.

Douglas, M. (1966) *Purity and Danger: an Analysis of the Concepts of Pollution and Taboo*. London: Routledge & Kegan Paul.

Dunlop, M. (1986) Is a science of caring possible? *Journal of Advanced Nursing*, 11, 661–70.

Dickenson, D. (2007) *Property in the Body*. NY: Cambridge University Press.

Eayrs, M.A. (1993) Time, trust and hazard: hairdressers' symbolic roles, *Symbolic Interaction*, 16, 19–37.

Emerson, R.M. and Pollner, M. (1976) Dirty work designations: their features and consequences in a psychiatric setting, *Social Problems*, 23, 243–54.

Folbre, N. and Nelson, J.A. (2000) For love or money – or both? *The Journal of Economic Perspectives*, 14, 4, 123–40.

Foner, N. (1994) *The Caregiving Dilemma*. Berkley, CA: University of California Press.

Foucault, M. (1997) Technologies of the self. In Rabinow, P. (ed.) *Michel Foucault: Ethics: Subjectivity and Truth*. New York: The New Press.

Frankenberg, R. (ed.) (1992) *Time, Health and Medicine*. London: Sage.

Gatta, M., Boushey, H. and Applebaum, E. (2009) High-touch and here-to-stay: future skill demands on low wage US service occupations, *Sociology*, 43, 5, 968–89.

George, M. (2008) Interactions in expert service work: demonstrating professionalism in personal training, *Journal of Contemporary Ethnography*, 37, 1, 108–31.

Giddens, A. (1990) *The Consequences of Modernity*. Cambridge: Polity Press.

Gimlin, D. (1996) Pamela's place: power and negotiation in the hair salon, *Gender and Society*, 10, 505–26.

Gimlin, D. (2007) What is Body Work? A review of the literature, *Sociology Compass*, 1, 1, 353–70.

Gimlin, D.L. (2002) *Body Work: Beauty and Self Image in American Culture*. Berkeley: University of California Press.

Glenn, E.N. (2001) The race and gender division in public reproductive labor. In Baldox, R., Koeber, C. and Kraft, K. (eds) *The Critical Study of Work*. Philadelphia: Temple University Press.

Graham, R. (2006) Lacking compassion – sociological analyses of the medical profession, *Social Theory and Health*, 4, 43–63.

Greer, S. (2008) Choosing paths in European Union health services policy, *Journal of European Social Policy*, 18, 3, 219–31.

Grosz, E. (1994) *Volatile Bodies: toward a Corporeal Feminism*. Indiana University Press, Bloomington.

Guevarra, A.R. (2006) Managing vulnerabilities and empowering migrant Filipina workers: the Philippines overseas employment program, *Social Identities*, 12, 523–41.

Gunaratnam, Y. (2001) 'We mustn't judge people . . . but': staff dilemmas in dealing with racial harassment amongst hospice service users, *Sociology of Health and Illness*, 23, 1, 65–84.

Gurney, C.M. and Means, R. (1993) The meaning of home in later life. In Arber, S. and Evandriou, M. (eds) *Ageing, Independence and the Life Course*. London: Jessica Kingsley.

Halford, S. and Leonard, P. (2003) Space and place in the performance of nursing identities, *Journal of Advanced Nursing*, 42, 2, 201–8.

Himmelweit, S. (2005) Can we afford not to care: prospects and policies. GeNet Working Paper 11, accessed 20.05.10 from http://www.genet.ac.uk/workpapers/GeNet205p11.pdf.

Hochschild, A. (1983) *The Managed Heart: Commercialisation of Human Feeling*. Los Angeles University of California Press.

Hochschild, A.R. (2003a) *The commercialization of intimate life: Notes from home and work*. Berkeley: University of California Press.

Hochschild, A.R. (2003b) Love and gold. In Ehrenreich, B and Hochschild, A.R. (eds) *Global Woman: Nannies, Maids and Sex Workers in the New Economy*. London: Granta Books.

Howarth, G. (1996) *Last Rites: the Work of the Modern Funeral Director*. New York: Baywood.

Howes, C. (2004) Upgrading California's home care workforce, *The State of California Labor 2004*: University of California Press. 71–105.

Jacoby, D. (2006) Caring about labour: an introduction, *Politics and Society*, 34, 1, 5–9.

James, N. (1989) Emotional labour: skill and work in the social regulation of feelings, *Sociological Review*, 37, 1, 15–42.

James, N. (1992) Care = organisation + physical labour + emotional labour, *Sociology of Health and Illness*, 14, 4, 488–509.

Kang, M. (2003) The managed hand: the commercialisation of emotion in Korean immigrantowned nail salons, *Gender and Society*, 17, 6, 820–39.

Kang, M. (2010) *The Managed Hand: Race, Class and Gender in Beauty Service Work*. Berkeley: University of California Press.

Katz, S. (2005) Spaces of age: snowbirds and the gerontology of mobility: the elderscapes of Charlotte County, Florida. In Katz, S. (ed.) *Cultural Aging: Life Course, Lifestyle and Senior Worlds*. Toronto: University of Toronto Press.

Korczynski, M. (2008) 'A Touching Story: the Body and the Enchanting Myth of Customer Sovereignty'. ESRC Seminar Series on Body Work, University of Kent, July. Available at http:// www2.warwick.ac.uk/fac/soc/sociology/rsw/current/body_work/seminars/3/seminar_3_-_korczynski

Lan, P.C. (2006) *Global Cinderellas: Migrant Domestics and Newly Rich Employers in Taiwan*. Durham, NC: Duke University Press.

Lawler, J. (1991) *Behind the Screens: Nursing, Somology and the Problem of the Body*. Melbourne: Churchill Livingstone.

Lawler, J. (1997) Knowing the body and embodiment: methodologies, discourses and nursing. In Lawler, J. (ed.) *The Body in Nursing*. Melbourne: Churchill Livingstone.

Lawton, J. (2003) Lay experiences of health and illness: past research and future agendas, *Sociology of Health and Illness*, Silver Anniversary Edition, 25, 3, 23–40.

Lee, O.F. and Davis, T.R.V. (2004) International patients: a lucrative market for US hospitals, *Health Marketing Quarterly*, 22, 1, 41–56.

Lee Treweek, G. (1994) Bedroom abuse: the hidden work in a nursing home, *Generations Review*, 4, 1, 2–4.

Lee-Treweek, G. (1996) Emotion work, order and emotional power in care assistant work. In James, V. and Gabe, J. (eds) *Health and the Sociology of the Emotions*. Oxford: Blackwell.

Lee-Treweek, G. (1998) Women, resistance and care: an ethnographic study of nursing auxiliary work, *Work, Employment and Society*, 11, 1, 47–63.

Lopez, S.H. (2006) Culture change management in long-term care: a shop-floor view, *Politics and Society*, 34, 1, 55–79.

Lowe, D.M. (1995) *The Body in Late Capitalist USA*. Durham, NC: Duke University Press.

Martin, E. (1994) *Flexible Bodies: Tracking Immunity in American Culture from the Days of Polio to the Age of AIDS*. Boston: Beacon.

McDonald, D. and Ruiters, G. (2006) *Rethinking Privatisation, Public Services Yearbook 2005/2006*. Amsterdam: Transnational Institute.

Macdonald, C. and Sirianni, C. (eds) (1996) *Working in the Service Society*. Philadelphia: Temple University Press.

McDowell, L. (2009) *Working Bodies: Interactive Service Employment and Workplace Identities*. Oxford: Wiley-Blackwell.

Moreira, T. (2004) Coordination and embodiment in the operating room, *Body and Society*, 10, 1, 109–29.

Nettleton, S., Burrows, R. and Watt, I. (2008) How do you feel doctor? An analysis of emotional aspects of routine professional medical work, *Social Theory and Health*, 6, 18–36.

Neysmith, S.M. and Aronson, J (1997) Working conditions in home care: negotiating race and class boundaries in gendered work, *International Journal of Health Services*, 27, 3, 479–99.

O'Connell Davidson, J. (1996) Sex tourism in Cuba, *Race and Class*, 38, 39–48.

Oerton, S. (2004) Bodywork boundaries: power, politics and professionalism in therapeutic massage, Gender, *Work and Organisation*, 11, 5, 544–65.

Player, S. and Leys, C. (2008) Commodifying health. In Huws, U. and Hermann, C. (eds) *The New Gold Rush*. London: Analytica Publications.

Parreñas, R.C. (2006) *The Forces of Domesticity: Filipina Migrants and Globalization*. New York: NYU Press.

Pfefferie, S.G. and Weinberg, D.B. (2008) Certified nurse assistants making meaning of direct care, *Qualitative Health Research*, 18, 7, 952–61.

Rakovski, C. and Price-Glynn, K. (2009) Caring labour, intersectionality and worker satisfaction: an analysis of the National Nursing Assistant Study (NNAS), *Sociology of Health and Illness*, 32, 3, 400–14.

Rankin, J. (2003) Patient satisfaction: knowledge for ruling hospital reform, *Nursing Inquiry*, 10, 1, 57–65.

Rapp, R. (1999) *Testing Women, Testing the Fetus*. New York and London: Routledge.

Razavi, S. (2007) The political and social economy of care in a developing context. *United Nations Research Institute for Social Development, Gender and Development Programme, paper 1*.

Rivas, L.M. (2003) Invisible labors: caring for the independent person. In Ehrenreich, B. and Hochschild, A.R. (eds) *Global Woman: Nannies, Maids and Sex Workers*. London: Granta Books.

Routasalo, P. (1999) Physical touch in nursing studies: a literature review, *Journal of Advanced Nursing*, 30: 843–50.

Rubinstein, R.L. (1989) The home environments of older people: a description of the psychosocial processes linking person to place, *Journal of Gerontology*, 44, 2, S45–53.

Sanders, T. (2004) A continuum of risk? The management of health, physical and emotional risks by female sex workers, *Sociology of Health and Illness*, 26, 5, 1–18.

Simonds, W. (2002) Watching the clock: keeping time during pregnancy, birth, and postpartum experiences, *Social Science and Medicine*, 55, 559–70.

Sixsmith, A. (1990) The meaning and experience of 'home' in later life. In Bytheway, B. and Johnson, J. (eds) *Welfare and the Ageing Experience*. Aldershot: Avebury.

Shilling, C. (1993) *The Body and Social Theory*. London: Sage.

Shilling, C. (2005) *The Body in Culture, Technology and Society*. London: Sage.

Smith, D. (1988) *The Everyday World as Problematic*. Boston: Northeastern University Press.

Snell, T. (2009) Home care services for older people in the United Kingdom, *Research Bites: Personal Social Services Research Unit Newsletter*, 6, spring/summer, 14–15.

Sointu, E. (2006) Healing bodies, feeling bodies: embodiment and alternative and complementary health practices, *Social Theory and Health*, 4, 3, 203–20.

Solari, C. (2006) Professionals and Saints: how immigrant careworkers negotiate gender identities at work, *Gender and Society*, 20, 3, 301–31.

Sweetman, P. (1999) Anchoring the (post) modern self: body modification, fashion and identity, *Body and Society*, 5, 2-3, 51–76.

Theodosius, C. (2008) *Emotional Labour in Health Care*. London: Routledge.

Twigg, J. (1999) The spatial ordering of care: public and private in bathing support at home, *Sociology of Health and Illness*, 21, 4, 381–400.

Twigg, J. (2000a) *Bathing – the Body and Community Care*. London: Routledge.

Twigg, J. (2000b) Carework as a form of bodywork, *Ageing and Society*, 20, 4, 389–411.

Twigg, J. (2006) *The Body in Health and Social Care*. Basingstoke: Palgrave.

Ungerson, C. (1983) Women and caring: skills, tasks and taboos. In Gamarnikow, E., Morgan, D., Purvis, J. and Taylorson, D. (eds) *The Public and the Private*. London: Heinemann.

Ungerson, C. (1993) Payment for caring: mapping a territory. In Deakin, N. and Page, R. (eds) *The Costs of Welfare*. Aldershot: Avebury.

Ungerson, C. (1999) Hybrid forms of work and care: the case of personal assistants and disabled people, *Work, Employment and Society*, 13, 4, 583–600.

Ungerson, C. (1997) Social politics and the commodification of care, *Social Politics*, 4, 362–81.

Waldby, C. (2000) Fragmented bodies, incoherent medicine, *Social Studies of Science*, 30, 3, 465–75.

Watson, N., McKie, L., Hughes, B., Hopkins, D. and Gregory, S. (2004) The potential for disability and feminist theorists to develop an emancipatory model, *Sociology*, 38, 2, 331–50.

Widding Isaksen, L. (2002a) Masculine dignity and the dirty body, *NORA*, 10, 3, 137–46.

Widding Isaksen, L. (2002b) Toward a sociology of (gendered) disgust: images of bodily decay and the social organization of care work, *Journal of Family Issues*, 23, 7, 791–811.

Witz, A., Warhurst, C. and Nickson, D. (2003) The labour of aesthetics and the aesthetics of organization, *Organization*, 10, 33–54.

Wolkowitz, C. (2002) The social relations of body work, *Work, Employment and Society*, 16, 3, 497–510.

Wolkowitz, C. (2006) *Bodies at Work*. London: Sage.

Wolkowitz, C. (2010) The body work economy of southeast Florida. Paper presented at the International Labour Process Conference, Rutgers, NJ. 15–17 March.

Wolkowitz, C. (2011) The organizational contours of body work. In Jeanes, E., Knights, D. and Yancey Martin, P. (eds) *Handbook of Gender, Work and Organization*. Chichester: Wiley-Blackwell.

Yeates, N. (2004) A dialogue with 'global care chain' analysis: nurse migration in the Irish context, *Feminist Review*, 79–95.

Zelizer, V. (2005) *The Purchase of Intimacy*. Princeton: Princeton University Press.

2

Time, space and touch at work: body work and labour process (re)organisation
Rachel Lara Cohen

Introduction

The present 'austerity' period is witnessing the emergence of a new political mantra: the realisation of 'efficiency savings' in health and social care without degradation of frontline services. This mantra shows naiveté about the work involved in delivering such services. Specifically, since health and social care services require workers to work on, with and sometimes inside the bodies of others, bodies are both the object of labour and the material of production. As this chapter will show, human bodies are a peculiarly intractable material of production. This intractability constrains the (re)organisation of work, especially labour rationalisation. Consequently, realising 'efficiency savings' is comparatively difficult and unlikely to occur without degradation in the treatment accorded to both workers and the bodies they work upon.

Increasingly, the sociology of health and illness has paid attention to embodiment (Corbin 2003, Williams 1996). There have also been excellent studies of the working lives and labour process experiences of health and social care providers, and of the consequences of structural (re)organisation for work in the sector (*cf.* Armstrong and Armstrong 2010, Doherty 2009). These two trends have, however, not been well integrated.[1] Sociological analysis of the labour process tends not to focus on patients' or workers' bodies, nor the requirement for bodily manipulation (Wolkowitz 2006: 14–6). Conversely, sociological analysis of the sick or medical body has paid little heed to the structural organisation and reorganisation of paid work on the body. This chapter suggests that conceptualising health and social care work as 'body work' (Gimlin 2007, Twigg 2000b, 2006, Wolkowitz 2002, 2006) enables us to bridge that gap. In so doing it also provides a lens through which to compare work in health and social care with work in other sectors.

Over 10 per cent of UK jobs involve 'body work': the touch, manipulation or physical constraint of bodies (see Table 1). These jobs are in expanding sectors: personal services and security, as well as health and social care. The workforce involved in 'body work' is therefore likely to increase over the foreseeable future. Consequently understanding the social organisation of body work is of growing importance to our ability to make sense of not only the health sector, but wider labour process conditions.

Conceptualising work as 'body work' also highlights an overlooked aspect of work: that bodies form the objects or materials of production for a range of jobs. Understanding the

Body Work in Health and Social Care, First Edition. Edited by Julia Twigg, Carol Wolkowitz, Rachel Lara Cohen and Sarah Nettleton.

Table 1 *Body labour, schedule and employment status. Labour Force Survey, Spring 2005*

	Schedule			Employment Status		Total
	Mean weekly hours	% Work Saturday	% Work Sunday	% Self-employed No employees	% Self-employed With employees	
Not body labour	32.8	25.6	15.5	9.9	2.9	25,171,130
Body labour*	30.0	44.8	36.4	9.0	3.2	2,932,679
Health professionals	40.6	29.0	19.2	9.3	23.4	223,994
Health associate professionals	29.9	47.5	44.8	2.2	0.4	613,011
Healthcare and related personal services	28.1	56.9	52.9	1.8	0.1	898,364
Childcare and related personal services	25.8	5.4	2.9	20.2	1.1	330,882
Therapists	25.7	12.0	6.1	30.1	2.8	139,739
Sports and fitness occupations	22.5	39.1	25.0	30.5	0.7	85,759
Hairdressers and beauty salon managers	32.1	81.2	3.8	27.4	52.6	30,919
Hairdressers and related occupations	26.4	66.6	6.1	37.8	6.6	189,914
Undertakers and mortuary assistants	30.5	21.2	18.8	8.6	1.8	16,173
Protective service officers	39.8	32.4	31.2	0.0	0.7	68,498
Protective service occupations	35.8	62.1	58.8	0.2	0.0	335,426

*'Body labour' occupations were selected at 3-digit level. Therefore where workers within these 2-digit occupational groups were judged as not directly involved in body labour (for example radiologists) they were coded as 'not body labour' and excluded from tallies for the occupational group (list of body labour by 3-digit occupation available on request from author). Reliance on standard occupational codes excludes some work, including work occurring on the interstices of legality such as sex work. Workers performing body labour in a second job are also omitted. A fuller version of this table was first produced by the author for a presentation to the ESRC seminar series on *Body Work* (see http://www.go.warwick.ac.uk/bodywork).

ways that working on bodies systematically delimits possibilities for the (re)organisation or rationalisation of the labour process – the ways in which these limits may be circumnavigated as well as why we may want them to be reinforced – suggests a novel and useful agenda for labour process analysis. It also provides a way of understanding why labour process (re)organisation in health and social care is difficult and contentious, and, why it rarely disappears from the socio-political agenda.

Organisation and reorganisation of the labour process

Notwithstanding professional or compassionate commitment to patients, work and employment in health and social care settings is played out on the same territory as other work in capitalism. This territory is marked by persistent, albeit not always predictable, conflict and constraint (Thompson and Smith 2010) and shaped by the imperative on capital to continually increase productivity and, to this end, engage in ongoing reorganisation and rationalisation of the labour process (Marx [1867] 1967). When organisations are in the public sector this imperative is somewhat altered, but increasingly the public sector is also subject to pseudo-market mechanisms, incorporating targets, audits and rewards for cost-cutting (Nettleton *et al.* 2008). Moreover, all workers, in public and not-for-profit as well as private organisations, sell their labour-power on the market, making it available only for a limited time (for instance from nine to five). Profit, or efficiency, therefore, depends on the output of these workers within this time period. This provides managers with the incentive to substitute labour with capital (often in the form of technology), extract the maximum effort and decrease the 'porosity of the working day' by minimising gaps or non-working time between tasks (Green 2001).

Whereas the above imperatives are general and abstract, any particular labour process, be it banking or nursing, involves specific tasks and specific constraints on the possibilities for (re)organisation. This chapter examines a space between these two poles. Three constraints on labour process organisation and reorganisation are identified. These are not general to all work, yet they span occupational divides as they are produced when work takes the bodies of others as its object. They are:

1. Rigidity in the ratio of workers to bodies-worked-upon limits the potential to increase capital-labour ratios or cut labour.
2. The requirement for co-presence and temporal unpredictability in demand for body work diminish the spatial and temporal malleability of the labour process.
3. The nature of bodies as a material of production – complex, unitary and responsive – makes it difficult to standardise, reorganise or rationalise work.

The main body of the chapter expands on these three constraints, exploring ways in which each might be overcome, in whole or in part. The chapter begins, however, by proposing a working definition of body work, and introducing the concept of 'body labour'.

Defining body work/body labour

Setting aside (for the moment) differences between paid and unpaid work, if body work is work 'on the bodies of others' what exactly is included? Possible responses include work on conscious bodies, work on live bodies, work on intact bodies,[2] work on body parts and work on bodily excretions. These responses are nested: work on conscious bodies necessarily encompasses all that follows – work on live, intact bodies, body parts and usually some excretions – but the reverse is not true; bodily excretions can be examined without encountering any live, intact bodies, or even body parts. In her overview of body work, Wolkowitz (2002) is ambiguous about how wide a conceptual net to cast. Her empirical examples involve direct and sustained contact with live, and usually conscious, bodies (nurses, care-workers, beauticians, sex-workers). She suggests, however, that body work might also encompass 'occupations that, even if they do not involve direct touching, deal with body fluids and wastes, [for example] hospital ward cleaners' (2002: 498). Notably, this includes those whose central purpose is the manipulation of body parts or emissions (for example, workers in a sperm bank or stem-cell scientists) *and* workers who encounter bodily emissions as debris out of place (hospital ward cleaners, but also any cleaner encountering a dirty toilet, human hairs, vomit or simply domestic dust). Such an expansive definition nicely highlights the centrality of others' physical bodies and their excretions to numerous jobs. Nonetheless, the treatment of bodies as a material object like any other, physical, malleable and ultimately divisible, obviates that which makes bodies a theoretically interesting object of labour and a fruitful subject for labour process analysis: that bodies are unitary, communicative *and* mindful. A clearly delineated conceptual boundary nonetheless remains elusive because, in practice, bodies slip between consciousness and unconsciousness, and work on live bodies may involve prone, unconscious, immobile or inarticulate bodies or bodies going between life and death. The definition adopted here is therefore pragmatic, rooted in a specific analytic goal – developing labour process analysis of body work.[3] It is: *body work involves the manipulation or touch of another's intact body.*

Body work has been used to describe *paid* work on the body of another (Gimlin 2007, Twigg 2000b, 2006, Wolkowitz 2002, 2006). In this chapter, however, I follow Kang (2010: 20–1), and by 'body work' refer to *all work on the body of another*, reserving 'body labour' for *body work that is sold for a wage or commodified*. This conceptually parallels the dichotomy made by Hochschild (1983: 7) between 'emotional work' and 'emotional labour', and therefore establishes a framework for analysing the interrelationship between emotional work/labour and body work/labour. The body work/labour distinction also recognises the difference between the work itself (the tasks) and the commodified form of these tasks. Whereas the tasks may be the same (for instance massaging a back), when these tasks are performed in commodified relations the end is not principally intrinsic or embodied but exterior and disembodied: profit or output targets rather than a relaxed back (although there are exceptions and qualifications). The following sections examine the social organisation of paid body work, or 'body labour'. The focus is health and social care, but examples from other body work sectors extend and situate the analysis, while contrasts with non-body work provide context.

The ratio of bodies, labour and capital

Body work is labour intensive. A single worker can only in exceptional circumstances work on multiple bodies concurrently: bodies are simply too large, complex and contrary. A nurse bandaging one patient cannot simultaneously take blood from another. A manicurist filing one client's fingernails cannot polish another's toenails. Notwithstanding worker dexterity, these scenarios are improbable. Accordingly, during the time that they work on any one body, the relationship between worker and body is minimally one-to-one. Where several workers work on a single body, for instance a surgical team clustered round a patient in an operating theatre, the relationship is many-to-one. Scale increases do not therefore directly produce efficiency gains; an increase in the number of bodies worked on requires a proportionate increase in labour. To cut costs, or increase profits, either the body must receive less attention (discussed below) or a division of labour introduced, with parts of the labour process assigned to lower-skilled, or at least lower-paid, workers. The latter has occurred over and again in health services (*cf.* Armstrong and Armstrong 2010: 149) as, for example, nurses are assigned tasks that were previously doctors' prerogative (Doherty 2009) and healthcare assistants take on nurses' tasks (Bach *et al.* 2009). It is also found in other fields. For example, larger hairdressing salons employ a high ratio of trainees to stylists. Paid less than half the wage of a stylist, trainees wash and blow-dry clients' hair, enabling (higher paid and higher skilled) hairstylists to 'see' more clients (Cohen 2005).

As simple tasks get sloughed off to lower-paid workers the number of workers attending to any one body increases. Although bodies remain unitary, this fractures institutional interactions with *the body* into multiple interactions, often each with a different body part at a different time. This undermines efforts to treat the body/person holistically; this is not the 'continuity of care' sought by patients, nor is it 'holistic nursing'. It also runs counter to the 'personalisation' that commercial sellers of body work foster (Toerien and Kitzinger 2007). Reorganisation involving labour substitution may therefore be a sign of patient/client relative disempowerment. Additionally, as each worker's embodied engagement with a patient's/client's body is reduced, their reliance on notes from co-workers or oral communication with the body-worked-upon increases. In this way an unintended by-product of labour substitution in body labour is increased reliance on workers' abilities to coax out, and offer, cogent verbal and written explanations of embodied states. Yet labour substitution simultaneously undermines workers' ability to build the relationships with patients/clients that would smooth these interactions.

Reducing the ratio of workers to bodies without labour substitution and without decreasing the attention paid to any one body may be possible where body labour is applied discontinuously; with gaps, or times when bodies are present but not being worked on. Such gaps occur, for example, while a patient waits with a thermometer under her tongue or a hairdressing client sits under the dryer while her perm 'takes'; patients/clients are in the workplace, but temporarily not being worked upon. Some gaps are brief; others, however, are sufficient for workers to move to work on another body. This facilitates either one-to-many or many-to-many relationships. A single worker or group of workers is able to work on multiple co-present bodies if not simultaneously then at least serially. Unfortunately, relying on labour process gaps to improve efficiency requires that workers can predict their periodicity and length. Bodies and their temporality are, however, frustratingly unpredictable (discussed further below).

Not all workers who do body labour spend all of their time doing it. Table 2 estimates the order of selected occupations on the basis of the proportion of total labour time spent engaged in body labour. At the top are jobs involving almost constant touch. A masseur spends the vast part of income-producing time physically engaged with a client's body; as is the case with a sex worker or manicurist. Turning to medical occupations, there is clearly a difference between a dentist and a General Practitioner. Whilst a dentist physically engages with every patient (Nettleton 1992: 14–16), a General Practitioner's interactions with some patients will be entirely discursive. Similarly, whereas home care workers are often called upon to perform general household tasks, including cleaning or even cooking (see England *et al.*, this book), care workers in residential homes spend more of the working day dealing with the bodily needs of residents, due to clearly delineated work roles and dedicated cooking and cleaning staff (Diamond 1992).

Table 2 *Body labour as estimated proportion of total labour*

100%	*Labour/capital reorganisation more difficult*
↑	Hairdresser, Masseur, Manicurist, Sex worker
	Dentist, Tattooist, Chiropractor
	Surgeon, Nurse, Orderly
	Paramedic, Residential care worker, Physiotherapist
	Home-care worker, Childcare worker, Nightclub bouncer
	General Practitioner, Yoga instructor,
	Psychiatrist, Airport security worker, Prison warden, Fire fighter
↓	Police officer, Football coach
0%	*Labour/capital reorganisation easier*

At the foot of Table 2 are occupations involving relatively infrequent touch or bodily manipulation. For example, an airport security guard sometimes, but infrequently, restrains or 'pats down' bodies. Similarly, a psychiatrist may occasionally conduct physical examinations, but spends significantly more time talking to patients, writing up notes or discussing cases with colleagues. Of course, the amount of body labour performed varies between psychiatric specialties, just as it does between security guards located in different environments.

In jobs where body labour is a smaller part of total labour (such as those at the foot of Table 2) or where the objects of body labour are present but do not require constant attention, it may become possible to lower the ratio of workers to bodies, thereby easing labour process reorganisation. It is not necessary to have one security guard for each body entering a nightclub or one care worker for every residential home occupant. The unpredictability of bodies means, however, that reductions in the worker-body ratio increase the likelihood that there are sometimes too few body workers. For example, if a nightclub fight breaks out requiring the restraint of several people, the need for body labour will suddenly spike. Similarly, several care-home residents may require toileting or to be taken to dinner simultaneously. Thus, critical in the organisation of body labour is *determining the balance between sporadically inactive labour and sporadically unattended bodies*. In some cases (for example, when someone is having a heart attack or a fire has broken out), making bodies wait is harmful, but in other cases (a medical check-up or a manicure), delay produces little more than patient/client frustration. This suggests that an important dimension in determining how easily body labour can be reorganised is the ability or not of the body- worked-upon to wait – or its relative neediness. Where bodies are needier, and where there are social arguments for addressing that need, sufficient labour must be employed to cover peaks. This means that during 'slack periods' labour is 'baggy', at work but not working. For instance, it is socially acceptable that sometimes fire fighters have little to do or that during (perhaps rare) quiet times hospital casualty ward staff will be unoccupied because their presence during rush times is essential.

Of course, the 'neediness' of bodies is not purely physical. It is also social, political and economic. As already suggested, where services are publically managed neediness is made concrete as public policy. This prioritises particular bodies. For example, the UK government has introduced strict 'waiting time targets' for cancer patients but not for other seriously ill patients, thus implicitly prioritising the former. In contrast, de-prioritisation of need and the normalisation of some bodies' discomfort is exposed by Diamond (1992), who details the habitual inattention care-home residents suffer:

Given the staff-resident ratio, it was deemed most efficient to have diapers put on many of the residents, so that their bodily cleaning could be attended to after the fact. By the time we reached some residents to change diapers, it might have been several hours after they had first called us. Residents had to learn to sit or lie in bed after an accident waiting for clean [liness] to be restored. (1992: 178, see also 87–8)

Lacking socio-economic power, residents are unable to characterise their bodily needs as important. Instead, in the context of labour shortages, residents are forced to 'learn' to cope with a situation most adults would find intolerable, effectively recalibrating bodily need.

The structural relationship between worker and body also affects the calculation of need. For instance, self-employed body workers, such as hairstylists, complementary and alternative medicine (CAM) practitioners and sports therapists, depend on repeat custom and, as such, have a structural incentive to be available when clients 'need' to see them, even at their own inconvenience. In contrast, waged workers are structurally independent from clients and less willing to accommodate (or legitimate) client need (Cohen 2010b).

Temporal and spatial malleability

Co-presence is tangential to much service work, a by-product of the need to communicate, transfer goods or display a corporate aesthetic in, respectively, business meetings, retail transactions and the cultural industry. Co-presence is, however, essential when the object of work is the physical manipulation of the body of a customer, client, or patient. Workers and bodies must inhabit the same time-spaces. This means that centralisation or wholesale off-shoring of body labour is unfeasible, notwithstanding pressures to cut costs by employing cheaper or fewer workers.[4] Regions have nonetheless emerged as both body work destinations (Argentina for plastic surgery; Eastern Europe for dentistry (Connell 2006); the Gulf Coast for care-homes) and as centres for body work training (whether Filipino nurses (Romina Guevarra 2006) or Cuban doctors (Feinsilver 2010)).

In non-body work service industries the need for co-presence has decreased with the expansion in remote or virtual interactions mediated by information and communication technologies (ICT). Similarly, attempts are being made to substitute co-present body labour for tele-presence; for instance, 'telemedicine' (Dyb and Halford 2009), which involves virtual links between patient and clinician or between multiple clinicians. Telemedicine enables cost-cutting, for example by centralising primary healthcare advice or reducing demand for home visits and out-of-hours doctors (Lattimer et al. 1998). It may be democratising, as expensive specialist medical expertise, such as surgeons, can be dispersed without dispersing specialists, although evidence for this remains scant. More pertinently, telemedicine barely reduces demand for geographically proximate body labour. Rather, advice-giving is separated off or body labour performed by cheaper workers with fewer specialist skills (the generalist or nurse practitioner, acting on the specialist's remote advice[5]). Hence, telemedicine hardly diminishes the demand for body labour. The success of this strategy may instead be the distillation of body labour in the health sector into 'manual work' in juxtaposition with 'mental' advice or direction. This is consequential for both patients and workers. Geographically remote surgeons may be more prone to objectifying patients (van Wynsberghe and Gastmans 2008: 4). Concomitantly, if it becomes denuded of decision-making capacity, the status of body work will further erode, intensifying the 'stigma' attached to close physical proximity with bodies (Isaksen 2002). This will only exacerbate current employment trends in body labour – which relies heavily on ultra-exploitable migrant female labour (Kang 2010, McDowell 2009). Meanwhile extension of the mental/ manual divide may increase the obstacles faced by patients who want control over their own physical care but whose embodied interactions are principally with workers lacking agency.

'Telecare' (Hibbert *et al*. 2003, Lopez and Domenech 2008) has achieved more reduction in the demand for body labour than telemedicine. Telecare often requires the patient (or body-worked-on) to self-monitor. Service users may operate an alarm themselves, sending information to a central location; alternatively the process may be entirely mechanised, for example, involving devices that automatically record blood pressure, and electronically trigger alarms. In both instances the requirement for a carer (paid or unpaid) to physically monitor the body is reduced. Nonetheless, once alerted, a worker is dispatched. Thus telecare does not eliminate the need for body labour but may make it possible to rationalise and allocate this from a centralised hub – with monitoring used to determine which bodies are (most) at need. Accordingly, it somewhat concentrates work without spatially centralising bodies-worked-upon. It also remains dependent upon an adequate bank of staff able to travel to bodies when required, something made difficult by the unpredictability of bodily need.

The intersection of the requirement for co-presence with the unpredictability of bodies' social and physical demands makes spatio-temporal organisation of body labour particularly tricky. As Twigg (2006: 128) notes, it is hard to schedule work on the body: 'care tasks cannot be accumulated and dealt with efficiently in one go: you cannot save up going to the toilet for a week and then do it just once. The body has its own timings.' This makes bodies a contrary material of production. Moreover, the biological unpredictability of bodies is exacerbated by consciousness and autonomous mobility (in contrast, unconscious or immobile bodies are less contrary and more easily 'trained', with a corpse the most manipulable of bodies). Accordingly, those who work on bodies often find it difficult to delimit working times and are disproportionately required to work outside the 'normal' working week. For example, as Table 1 shows, workers who do body labour are about 1.75 times as likely as other workers to work on Saturdays and over twice as likely to work on Sundays.

A closer examination of weekend working hints at several distinct patterns for the temporality of body labour. The first encompasses workers engaged in bodily adornment: hairdressers, beauticians, tattooists and, to a lesser extent, personal trainers. These workers must 'enchant' (Korczynski 2005) and temporally accommodate their 'customers'. As such, almost all workers performing body labour for adornment work on Saturdays. Since the 'need' for adornment is unlikely to arise with extreme unexpectedness or urgency most of these workers do manage one weekend day, Sunday, without work. In contrast, workers responsible for the health or control of bodies – nurses, emergency room doctors, paramedics and care assistants, as well as prison warders and security staff – are almost as likely to work on Sundays as Saturdays. For instance, over half of the workers classified as 'healthcare and related personal services' work on each of Saturday (57%) and Sunday (53%). The figures for 'protective service occupations' are similar (62% and 59%). Three types of body worker are, however, under substantially less pressure to extend their working time into the weekend. The first is undertakers. Working on dead bodies, undertakers are able to exercise some schedule and workplace control. The second is child-care providers. This is an interesting case in which workers' body labour is a direct (paid) substitute for unpaid (usually familial) body work. As such, the temporal need for the former depends on the employment or other commitments of the latter. Consequently, child-care workers' hours closely coincide with the 'normal' working week. The third group with little pressure to extend their working hours comprises workers providing 'non-urgent' medical care, including, for example, salaried primary care physicians, district nurses, dentists and therapists. Non-urgent medical care occupies a quite specific position with regard to the temporality of social need, on the one hand, 'non-urgent' and so not provided around the clock. On the other hand, it is accorded sufficient social importance that patients are (usually) able to secure leave from employment or education and schedule appointments during 'normal' working hours, thereby allowing this group of body workers to enjoy relatively regular working hours.[6]

If the temporal contrariness of bodies produces pressure to extend hours, it also makes it difficult to distribute work evenly across the working day. A constant work pace requires bodies be ready at the place and time that workers finish work on a previous body. Without bodies to work on, time hangs baggily. Thus one of the features of much body work is moments, even hours, of baggy time, followed by periods of intensive work. When rewards for labour are based on time at work (for example, hourly pay) baggy time is costly for employers. Thus there is an incentive to reorganise body work in order to overcome this and decrease the 'porosity of the working day'. In some respects this drive is no different to that found more generally (Green 2001). However, as discussed below, the elimination of baggy time may have additional consequences and be especially tricky when bodies are the material of production being reorganised.

One way that a continuous stream of work can be achieved and baggy time eliminated is through the spatial concentration of 'needy' bodies. Residential care homes are exemplary here: bodies are proximate and the productive use of gaps in bodily need is possible. Thus Lopez (2007: 235) describes care workers leaving residents alone on the toilet (despite formal rules prohibiting this), in order to use the brief temporal in-betweens to attend to other residents. Care home residents are, however, not only clustered but also lack mobility and are, as suggested above, relatively powerless. Their powerlessness is additionally important to the temporal management of body labour. Thus hard-pressed residential care-workers systematically ignore residents' requests to sleep late in the morning, in order to manage the intense work demands involved in getting all residents up and to breakfast on time (Diamond 1992: 77–9). In a similar vein, self-employed mobile hairstylists may seek out elderly clients, who are immobile and dependent, precisely in order to gain control of their schedules and the spatial and temporal organisation and ordering of work (Cohen 2010a). Thus, as the dependence or powerlessness of the body-worked-upon increases, temporal control shifts to the worker and, when the worker is an employee, the employing organisation.

Where it is not possible to reorganise the working day or spatially concentrate bodies-worked-upon, self-employment, especially own-account work or 'self-employment without employees', is common. Since the hours of work of the self-employed worker are not valued on the market, there is no requirement to recoup a specific hourly return. Consequently, although 'baggy time' may slow down the earnings of own-account-workers, thus requiring additional hours to achieve a given return (or 'self-exploitation'), it does not make labour costs uneconomic, as it would if body labour were performed by hourly paid waged employees. Accordingly, there has been relatively little concentration of private capital in body work sectors and, as Table 1 shows, a proliferation of self-employment in body labour occupations in the UK outside the two large nationalised sectors (health and protection). The dominant role played by large scale capital in the US health sector, for instance, in Health Maintenance Organisations (HMOs), initially contradicts this. Yet even in the US, sites of body labour have undergone relatively little concentration. For instance, a study of US private physicians found that 47 per cent practised solo or with one other physician, with a further 35 per cent based in practices of three to nine physicians (Casalino *et al.* 2003). Generally, HMOs have exerted control over body labour via contracting rather than direct employment relationships. Partial explanation for this may be found in the difficulty of consistently utilising labour.

Standardisation and reorganisation

Bodies' temporal unpredictability is indicative of the difference between body time and the abstract clock time of capitalism (Adam 1993). Bodies are not unique in adhering to a temporality at odds with capitalist production. Indeed, related arguments have been made about other organic materials, perhaps most persuasively by Susan Mann (1990) in an examination of the (relatively) slow entry of capital into agricultural production. In agriculture, however, capital investment has increasingly standardised production times and inputs, minimising the impact of organic phenomena, from seasonality to insect predators. This section examines the extent to which such standardisation and rationalisation of bodies has been able to remake bodies as predictable materials of production, including refitting body time to capitalist time.

Standardisation is desired because it enables the predictable allocation of resources. This facilitates a division of labour whereby parts of the process (and eventually perhaps the whole process) are performed by cheaper (unskilled) labour or are mechanised, increasing efficiency and profitability. Standardisation alone may not however improve efficiency. A case in point is the standardisation of appointment times common to upmarket hair salons. These, for example, specify that a restyle must occupy an hour-long appointment. This is sufficient time to accomplish most new styles at a measured pace, thereby indicating the 'quality' of the service, while allowing time for stylists to suggest extra treatments and products (possibly earning commission). Since, however, the complexity of a restyle and the thickness, texture and condition of hair vary there is actually little standard about these timings. This means that should clients have thin hair or request easy restyles, workers resort to 'drying' or 'styling' hair that is already thoroughly dry and styled simply to fill time (Cohen 2005). This is a form of 'standardising up' – setting standard timings at maximums. It is notable that standardising up, which appears a paradoxical way to rationalise labour use, since it reduces labour efficiency, occurs primarily where 'service' premiums are sought. Thus it indicates the relative power of the body-worked-upon in this sector and the related requirement to represent body labour in terms of both quality and value.

Caesarean birth provides a contrasting instance of bodily standardisation, and one which demonstrates the intersection of temporal standardisation with definite structures of employment and compensation. The World Health Organization estimates that caesareans are medically 'appropriate' in between 5 and 15 per cent of births (Althabe and Belizán 2006: 1472) yet all OECD countries except the Netherlands have rates exceeding this maximum (MacDorman *et al.* 2008: 296). Rates in Latin America are especially high. Moreover, a study of eight Latin American countries (Villar *et al.* 2006) found that 'the proportion of caesarean delivery was always higher in private hospitals'. For example, in Brazil, caesarean rates in private clinics were as high as 90 per cent, with, 'higher caesarean delivery rates mostly due to an increase in elective caesarean delivery'. The times and personnel involved in performing caesareans also differ between private and public hospitals. For instance, one comparative study showed that deliveries in a public clinic were performed by the doctor on duty, whereas in a private clinic 96 per cent of deliveries were performed by the doctor who had performed prenatal care. At the public clinic deliveries occurred on all seven days of the week at relatively similar rates; at the private clinic only 10 per cent of deliveries occurred on Saturdays and 5 per cent on Sundays. At the public clinic deliveries were equally likely over the four quarters of the day; at the private clinic only 10.4 per cent of deliveries occurred during the night (0:00 to 5:59) with the greatest number (36%) in the shift immediately prior to this (18:00 to 23:59) (de Almeida *et al.* 2008: 2911).[7] These figures describe a gradual standardisation of body time within (especially) private medicine. In this case a medical intervention, elective caesarean, is used to overcome the temporal unpredictability of childbirth despite costs to the bodies being standardised: an increased risk to the health of mother and foetus. Generally, caesareans are compensated at the same rate as natural birth, but are quicker and can be planned. Thus, 'doctors save much time and fit in many more activities by scheduling caesareans' (McCallum 2005: 232).[8] Employment relations and the wider structures of social healthcare also influence incentives for, and the form taken by, standardisation. For example, private prenatal healthcare in Brazil uses a 'single named obstetrician model'. Care is personalised and doctors have an interest in producing and retaining a 'clientele'. Because a single doctor is given sole responsibility for each patient's obstetric work, care must fit within this doctor's working (and waking) hours. This is only realisable by exerting temporal control over patients' bodies (Murray and Elston 2005: 715).[9]

A recent Royal College of Physicians report (2010) revealed another medical intervention aimed at the standardisation of bodies: the fitting of artificial feeding tubes. The report caused quite a stir in the UK media. Most news coverage concentrated on anecdotal evidence of residential care homes making it a condition of admittance that residents be fitted with feeding tubes, 'because staff shortages mean there is not enough time for conventional feeding' (Lister 2010). Artificial feeding tubes enable feeding to occur efficiently and whenever required. Feeding tubes also circumvent two otherwise time-consuming and unpredictable body labour activities: the intensive palliative support necessary to overcome temporary swallowing difficulties and ongoing mealtime support. Since such mealtime body labour may be required by several residents simultaneously, it is especially difficult for workers to manage. The fitting of feeding tubes is thus a 'rational' solution; a way of physically and temporally standardising and managing bodies. As US studies have found, it is one that is also most common where there are staff shortages and care homes are run on a for-profit basis (*cf.* Lopez *et al.* 2010, Mitchell *et al.* 2003). When the Royal College of Physicians report hit the headlines, it was, however, greeted with outrage, with articles appearing across the print and broadcast media highlighting that, 'the technique [artificial feeding] risks infections and also deprives patients of the pleasure of taste, and social interaction that come with normal eating' (Lister 2010). As this discussion, from *The Times* newspaper, indicates, bodies are not and cannot be treated as a material of production, like any other. Feeding is understood as more than a simple biological requirement to be managed 'efficiently'. The example therefore demonstrates both the ongoing attempts to mechanically standardise bodies and the ongoing resistance to this.

Body work sectors outside health and social care have also seen attempts to mechanise and standardise interactions with bodies. For example, scanning machines at building entrances automate bodily searches, which would otherwise require a security guard performing a 'pat down'. Coin-operated massage chairs, common in airport lounges, obviate the need for a masseur, while, mechanical seat and pillow 'massagers' are increasingly popular retail items. Yet, unlike a trained masseur, mechanical massagers cannot easily adapt to different bodies. Safety requires settings appropriate for the frailest of bodies, meaning bodies cannot be vigorously pummelled. Similarly, since automated body technologies are designed for the 'average body', they inevitably fit some bodies poorly, as illustrated by a customer review for a 'shiatsu massager' available at British retailer Argos.com:

> I am quite tall and would have preferred it if the massage could have gone a little bit higher, it stopped between my shoulder blades and I wanted it to keep going all the way to the back of my neck.

The above highlights the difficulties involved in producing a standardised mechanical device suitable for all bodies. An ill-fitting massager may be uncomfortable, but in other bodily interactions, for example a dental extraction, misfit could be bloody. Unsurprisingly, therefore, wholesale standardisation and mechanisation has made few inroads into body labour.

More often standardisation is piecemeal, barely apparent and subject to little resistance. For instance across body work sectors and in manifold ways bodies are prepared and made predictable in preparation for being worked upon. This frequently disempowers and, as Wolkowitz notes, is designed to constrain the body-worked-upon:

> Even when the worked-on-body is not physically weakened through disability, old age or the humiliation of double incontinence, it is frequently anaesthetised, supine or naked, or rendered immobile by gown or facial mud pack, making it difficult for the patient, customer or client to just get up and leave (Wolkowitz 2006: 163–4).

The foregoing examples of standardisation describe in various guises the enforced transformation of the body-worked-upon in order to produce a more predictable and malleable material of production. Collectively these might be typified as *standardisation by transformation*. A second set of practices also involves standardisation, but not transformation. Collectively, they may be characterised as *standardisation by selection*. Standardisation by selection can also take various forms, but because it does not require remaking the body, it has faced considerably less resistance than standardisation by transformation. The first selection point is body type. It is notable that a lot of body labour is delimited by the age, sex or other physical or social attribute, of the bodies-worked-upon (old bodies, babies' bodies, female bodies), which in turn diminishes both the physical and social variability of the work. For instance, some branches of medicine are defined by the age of the body-worked-upon (geriatrics, paediatrics) whereas other specialties involve only female bodies (obstetrics and gynaecology). Similarly, prison guards tend to work with only male or only female bodies; most sex workers work primarily with men; many hair salons specialise in men's or women's or afro-Caribbean hair; while childcare and care home workers work with young and old bodies respectively. A second form of standardisation by selection involves focusing on a single body part, whether hair, eyes, nose, feet or spine. Finally, most body workers carry out specific and limited procedures on those body parts with which they are concerned. For example, an optometrist and an ophthalmologist will approach and engage with the eye differently. Equally, a manicurist and podiatrist may both specialise on feet but have a different focus.

The result of standardisation by selection is that the live body is effectively divided into parts and functions rather than being treated as an organic and social entity. As such, it exacerbates tendencies towards dividing the body that emerge from the use of a division of labour to cheapen labour (discussed above). That bodies-worked-upon (patients or clients), recognise the medical and social limitations of this is seen in recurring pleas for 'joined up' health services, which are, effectively, calls for the recombination of the body-worked-upon. There seems, however, little evidence that these will be heeded, partly because standardisation by selection increases the speed with which bodies can be assessed and managed by limiting the number of, and variation in, the bodily functions of concern. It also facilitates the relatively cheap production of specialist workers and, increasingly, stand-alone centres with extensive knowledge in one body type, part, process or aesthetic, but little knowledge or interest in others. Perhaps unsurprisingly, many of the inroads made by private companies into the UK's National Health Service depend upon this form of standardisation; contracting to perform a single common operation (such as cataract surgery) at high volume.

Standardisation by selection appears less brutal than standardisation by transformation; neither, however, recognises the body as holistic, nor as mindful. This highlights a final tension: when body work takes the form of body labour – paid work on the body of another – there is inexorable pressure to standardise and reorganise the labour process. While some standardisation by selection is perhaps inevitable, standardisation is inherently dehumanising, because human beings are not standard, not temporally and not physically. Yet whether (and how) resistance to standardisation from the body-worked-upon, in the form of patient, user or client groups, may intersect with and potentially reinforce resistance to labour standardisation and deskilling on the part of body workers, remains to be seen.

Discussion

Body labour does not involve a single set of practices, nor a single set of workers or bodies-worked-upon. Despite the diversity of forms taken by body labour, there are, however, important commonalities. Amongst these is a set of labour process constraints that occur when work takes the human body as its object. These constraints arise out of the intersection between the dynamics of capitalist employment relations and the properties of the body-worked-upon. Bodies are complex, labour intensive materials to work with. They are indivisible and located. They do not keep to industrial time and are frustratingly contrary. They are also varied, physically and socially. Lastly, they can respond in multiple ways: physically (hitting out, clenching teeth, walking away, following or not following instructions), verbally (complaining or with geniality) and, most uniquely, collectively (in social or political movements, or through the state). As such, bodies-worked-upon can demand more or different body labour be applied and direct or resist body labour.

Different bodies are differently able to make demands for, or resist, body labour. Their ability to do this depends on their physical power or frailty, nakedness or exposure (Twigg 2000a). The power to demand or resist body labour also depends upon the structural relationship between body worker and body-worked-upon. This relationship may (a) be mediated by various other actors. For example, care work is funded by the state, co-ordinated by a private organization/employer, carried out by an employee, negotiated with a relative, and performed on a body. Alternatively, the relationship may (b) involve the body-worked-upon and body worker only. For example, there is a direct and unmediated relationship between the self-employed masseur and her client; as there is between the disabled employer of a home care worker. In both (b) scenarios the body worker is directly financially dependent upon the body-worked-upon, albeit employed within different formal structures (self-employed and employee). In scenario (a) the body worker's income is entirely independent of the body-worked-upon; yet both may be structurally disempowered vis-à-vis a private employer, the state or other actors. These scenarios highlight variation in the distribution of power, dependence and interdependence between body-worked-upon and body worker. Finally, the power of body-worked-upon vis-à-vis body worker depends on the relative socio-economic position of each. While, within the close confines of body labour, gendered, racialised and sexualised power structures can become tangible (Kang 2010, Wolkowitz 2006).

For sociologists of work and the labour process, examination of body labour serves a reminder that the concrete form taken by workers' labour matters. Partly because this sets limits on capital's capacity to transform the labour process at will. Body labour is not necessarily better, nor worse, than other work. It is, however, perhaps uniquely difficult to rationalise, not least because transformations of the labour process directly impact on the body-worked-upon. In this context struggles between the capital and workers over labour process (re)organisation cannot but include other actors: first, the body-worked-upon, but also the state, whether as regulator or employer of last resort. In this context struggles over labour-use, the reorganisation of the day, or the standardisation of the body are not predictable. Their resolution will depend upon a series of intersecting struggles, over issues as diverse as resource allocation, regulatory frameworks, working conditions and bodily violability, and will most likely involve the collective organisation of both body workers and bodies-worked-upon (in patient or user groups).

The organisational 'constraints' discussed herein, may or may not be problematic when body work is performed in extra-economic social relations, subject to different rationalities and temporal logics. For instance, when body work is carried out by a friend or a family member, gaps between tasks may not signify 'inefficient time use', but rather facilitate conversation, TV-watching or other activities of the life-world. Governments readily understand and exploit this (albeit perhaps implicitly) and increasingly provide social welfare in the form of direct payments to family members to provide care (Simonazzi 2009) thereby circumventing problems associated with commodified, especially waged, body labour.[10] It might be the case that this will in turn extend pressures to standardise and reorganise body work to extra-work spaces and social relations, concomitantly extending the systematic transformation and fragmentation of the body-worked-upon.

Acknowledgements

I am grateful to Sarah Nettleton, Julia Twigg and Carol Wolkowitz for their comments and support, to the anonymous reviewers for their helpful suggestions and Simon Kirwin for his editing. Many of the ideas presented here were developed during the ESRC funded *Body Work Seminar Series*. I would like to thank everyone who participated in these seminars.

Notes

1   Nettleton *et al.* (2008) are an exception.
2   Intact body is contrasted here with the separated body (or separable body parts and excretions), not the 'disabled' or 'damaged' body.
3   Where the focus is body work as 'dirty work' (Isaksen 2002, McDowell 2009: 167–74, Twigg 2000b, 2006: 136–7) a broader definition (including work on bodily emissions), may be preferable, as this nicely links the 'dirtiness' of work on bodies, especially messy bodies, to demeaning and distasteful cleaning work.
4   Centralisation may have benefits beyond cost-cutting. For instance, centralisation of infrequent surgical procedures facilitates skill acquisition and resource concentration, potentially improving patient outcomes. Changes in labour allocation do not however simply reflect 'technical' advan-

tages (such as surgical effectiveness). They also reflect economic or other social logics; logics which determine the parameters by which 'technical advantage' is calculated.

5   Telesurgery, where a distant surgeon is sole surgeon, may become more common as robotics advance. This however requires massive development and dissemination of technology and, critically, improved telecommunications reliability.

6   The political, and economic, strength and professional organisation of primary physicians and other non-urgent care providers may have contributed to the construction of this model of social need.

7   A US study similarly found that caesarean rates were highest where women had private insurance (Stafford 1990). Therefore these patterns of medical intervention into labour are not confined to Latin America.

8   There is relatively little evidence of women choosing caesareans for non-medical reasons despite widespread media hyperbole about being 'too posh to push' (McCallum 2005, Weaver *et al.* 2007).

9   A UK move to make a single midwife responsible for a woman throughout her pregnancy was quickly found to have 'such dire implications for the predictability of midwives' working hours . . . that it made recruitment and retention of midwives increasingly difficult' (Wolkowitz 2006: 163). This exemplifies the problems of individualised body work.

10 Recent Conservative Party (UK) proposals for a 'Big Society', where non-waged (voluntary) labour is used to provide social care and, potentially, healthcare can similarly be read as an attempt to circumvent inflexibilities in the absolute quantity of labour required to deliver these services.

References

Adam, B. (1993) Within and beyond the time economy of employment relations: conceptual issues pertinent to research on time and work, *Social Science Information*, 32, 163–84.

Althabe, F. and Belizán, J.M. (2006) Caesarean section: the paradox, *The Lancet*, 368, 1472–3.

Armstrong, P. and Armstrong, H. (2010) Contradictions at work: struggles for control in Canadian health care, *Socialist Register*, 46, 145–67.

Bach, S., Kessler, I. and Heron, P. (2009) Nursing a grievance? The role of healthcare assistants in a modernized National Health Service, *Gender, Work and Organization*, article first published online: 20 December 2009.

Casalino, L.P., Devers, K.J, Lake, T.K., Reed, M. and Stoddard, J.J. (2003) Benefits of and barriers to a large medical group practice in the United States, *Archives of Internal Medicine*, 163, 1958–64.

Cohen, R.L. (2005) Styling labor: work relations and the labor process in hairstyling. Doctoral Thesis, Sociology, UCLA, Los Angeles.

Cohen, R.L. (2010a) Rethinking 'mobile work': boundaries of space, time and social relations in the working lives of mobile hairstylists, *Work, Employment and Society*, 24, 65–84.

Cohen, R.L. (2010b) When it pays to be friendly: employment relationships and emotional labour in hairstyling, *Sociological Review*, 58, 197–218.

Connell, J. (2006) Medical tourism: sea, sun, sand and . . . surgery, *Tourism Management*, 27, 6, 1093–1100.

Corbin, J.M. (2003) The body in health and illness, *Qualitative Health Research*, 13, 256–67.

de Almeida, S., Bettiol, H., Barbieri, M.A., da Silva, A.A.M. and Ribeiro, V.S. (2008) Significant differences in cesarean section rates between a private and a public hospital in Brazil, *Cadernos de Saúde Pública*, 24, 2909–18.

Diamond, T. (1992) *Making Gray Gold: Narratives of Nursing Home Care*. Chicago: University of Chicago Press.

Doherty, C. (2009) A qualitative study of health service reform on nurses' working lives: learning from the UK National Health Service (NHS). *International Journal of Nursing Studies*, 46, 1134–42.

Dyb, K. and Halford, S. (2009) Placing globalizing technologies: telemedicine and the making of difference, *Sociology*, 43, 232–49.

Feinsilver, J. (2010) Cuban health politics at home and abroad, *Socialist Register*, 46, 216–39.

Gimlin, D. (2007) What is 'body work'? A review of the literature, *Sociology Compass*, 1, 353–70.

Green, F. (2001) It's been a hard day's night: the concentration and intensification of work in late twentieth century Britain, *British Journal of Industrial Relations*, 39, 53–80.

Hibbert, D., Mair, F.S., Angus, R.M., May, C., Boland, A., *et al.* (2003) Lessons from the implementation of a home telecare service, *Journal of Telemedicine and Telecare*, 9, 55–6.

Hochschild, A.R. (1983) *The Managed Heart: Commercialization of Human Feeling*. Berkeley: University of California Press.

Isaksen, L.W. (2002) Masculine dignity and the dirty body, *NORA – Nordic Journal of Feminist and Gender Research*, 10, 137–46.

Kang, M. (2010) *The Managed Hand: Race, Gender, and the Body in Beauty Service Work*. Berkeley: University of California Press.

Korczynski, M. (2005) The point of selling: capitalism, consumption and contradictions, *Organization*, 12, 69–88.

Lattimer, V., George, S., Thompson, F., Thomas, E., Mullee, M., *et al.* (1998) Safety and effectiveness of nurse telephone consultation in out of hours primary care: randomised controlled trial, *British Medical Journal*, 317, 1054–9.

Lister, S. (2010) *Care home patients given feeding tubes 'to save on staffing', The Times*. London: News International.

Lopez, S.H. (2007) Efficiency and the fix revisited: informal relations and mock routinisation in a nonprofit nursing home, *Qualitative Sociology*, 30, 225–47.

López, D. and Domènech, M. (2008) Embodying autonomy in a home telecare service, *Sociological Review*, 56, 181–95.

Lopez, R.P., Amella, E.J., Strumpf, N.E., Teno, J.M. and Mitchell, S.L. (2010) The influence of nursing home culture on the use of feeding tubes, *Archives of Internal Medicine*, 170, 83–88.

MacDorman, M.F., Menacker, F. and Declercq, E. (2008) Cesarean birth in the United States: epidemiology, trends, and outcomes, *Clinics in Perinatology*, 35, 293–307.

Mann, S. (1990) *Agrarian Capitalism in Theory and Practice*. Chapel Hill: University of North Carolina Press.

Marx, K. ([1867] 1967) *Capital*, volume I. New York: New World.

McCallum, C. (2005) Explaining caesarean section in Salvador da Bahia, Brazil, *Sociology of Health and Illness*, 27, 2, 215–42.

McDowell, L. (2009) *Working Bodies: Interactive Service Employment and Workplace Identities*. Chichester: Wiley-Blackwell.

Mitchell, S.L., Teno, J.M., Roy, J., Kabumoto, G. and Mor, V. (2003) Clinical and organizational factors associated with feeding tube use among nursing home residents with advanced cognitive impairment, *Journal of the American Medical Association*, 290, 73–80.

Murray, S.F. and Elston, M.A. (2005) The promotion of private health insurance and its implications for the social organisation of healthcare: a case study of private sector obstetric practice in Chile, *Sociology of Health and Illness*, 27, 6, 701–21.

Nettleton, S. (1992) *Power, Pain and Dentistry*. Buckingham: Open University Press.

Nettleton, S., Burrows, R. and Watt, I. (2008) Regulating medical bodies? The consequences of the 'modernisation' of the NHS and the disembodiment of clinical knowledge, *Sociology of Health and Illness*, 30, 3, 333–48.

Romina Guevarra, A. (2006) Managing vulnerabilities and empowering migrant Filipina workers: the Philippines' Overseas Employment Program, *Social Identities*, 12, 523–41.

Royal College of Physicians (2010) *Oral feeding difficulties and dilemmas: a guide to practical care, particularly towards the end of life*. London.

Simonazzi, A. (2009) Care regimes and national employment models, *Cambridge Journal of Economics*, 33, 211–32.

Stafford, R.S. (1990) Cesarean section use and source of payment: an analysis of California hospital discharge abstracts, *American Journal of Public Health*, 80, 313–15.

Thompson, P. and Smith, C. (2010) Working life: renewing labour process analysis. In Grugulis, I., Lloyd, C., Smith, C. and Warhurst, C. (eds) *Critical Perspectives on Work and Employment*. London: Palgrave.

Toerien, M. and Kitzinger, C. (2007) Emotional labour in action: navigating multiple involvements in the beauty salon, *Sociology*, 41, 645–62.

Twigg, J. (2000a) *Bathing: the Body and Community Care*. London: Routledge.

Twigg, J. (2000b) Carework as a form of bodywork, *Ageing and Society*, 20, 389–411.

Twigg, J. (2006) *The Body In Health and Social Care*. Basingstoke: Palgrave.

van Wynsberghe, A. and Gastmans, C. (2008) Telesurgery: an ethical appraisal, *Journal of Medical Ethics*, 34, e22.

Villar, J., Valladares, E., Wojdyla, D., Zavaleta, N., Carroli, G., *et al.* (2006) Caesarean delivery rates and pregnancy outcomes: the 2005 WHO global survey on maternal and perinatal health in Latin America, *The Lancet*, 367, 1819–29.

Weaver, J.J., Statham, H. and Richards, M. (2007) Are there unnecessary cesarean sections? Perceptions of women and obstetricians about cesarean sections for nonclinical indications *Birth*, 34, 32–41.

Williams, S.J. (1996) The vicissitudes of embodiment across the chronic illness trajectory, *Body and Society*, 2, 23–47.

Wolkowitz, C. (2002) The social relations of body work. *Work, Employment and Society*, 16, 497–510.

Wolkowitz, C. (2006) *Bodies at Work*. London: Sage.

3

Managing the body work of home care
Kim England and Isabel Dyck

Introduction

> I'm an attendant. We do anything the client needs to have done. It's very different,
> varies from client to client, it's mainly personal care. So everything – you get them up,
> dressed, showered, bed bath, catheter care, bowel treatment, anything; shaving,
> whatever the person needs (Alexa, attendant of Sarah, who has MS).[1]

Alexa, who works for a non-profit, publicly funded home healthcare agency in Ontario, was responding to a question about what sorts of tasks her job involves. As an attendant providing personal care, Alexa's occupation can be categorised as body work – jobs that involve intimate work done directly on other people's bodies. Alexa travels to her clients' homes to provide that care. Sarah is one of five clients Alexa cares for over the course of a week. She sees 50-year-old Sarah three mornings a week for two hours.

At various points during our lives we are each dependent on the care of others. For many, that dependency comes with old age, chronic illness or disability. In some instances, the care is provided by a family member or a friend; in other cases, it comes from a paid care worker such as a Registered Nurse (RN), a Registered Practical Nurse (RPN) or a Personal Support Worker (PSW). Sometimes, the care is given by a combination of both, as is the case with Sarah, whose primary caregiver is her husband, Andy, and in addition to Alexa, is visited by Celia, a PSW, and Sandy, an RPN. Glenda and Robert are also in Ontario's home care system, they too are cared for by family members and paid care workers. In this chapter we draw on the experiences of these three care recipients, their family caregivers and their paid care workers in our exploration of the management of the material micro-practices of body work and care relationships in home care. Recent extensive restructuring of health and social care services means the home is increasingly a key site in the landscape of long-term care and is a space where meanings of both home and care must be negotiated. Our emphasis on the intimate care of the body points up the diverse dynamics of care work through which caregivers, care recipients and homespace are constituted.

In the first section of the chapter, we discuss the conceptual framing. We then provide contextual material on the restructuring of home care in Canada, where the study on which we report was conducted, and we describe the study methods. The main themes emerging from the qualitative data are discussed in building our analysis of the active co-constitution

Body Work in Health and Social Care, First Edition. Edited by Julia Twigg, Carol Wolkowitz, Rachel Lara Cohen and Sarah Nettleton.

of body work through the dynamics and management of the caregiver/care recipient relationship. We argue that the micro-practices of care in the home are shaped by a complex interweaving of regulatory mechanisms associated with healthcare reform and the affective dimensions of intimate care, which suggests the need for new ways of understanding body work in contemporary landscapes of care.

Care as body work

As Diemut Bubeck (1995: 160) states, 'Care is a deeply human practice'. Each of us will receive and provide care over the course of our lives, and human life is deeply implicated in the inter-dependence of people who need and give care. There is a burgeoning literature on theorising and expanding the concept of care, including using it as a broad framework for making moral, political and policy decisions (see for example: Tronto 1993, Sevenhuijsen 1998, Kittay 1999, Held 2006). In this chapter we use 'care' to describe the varied activities associated with the daily care of the elderly and people with illnesses and disabilities, following Bubeck's definition of care. She opts for a 'restrictive definition of care as an activity' specifically 'meeting the needs of one person by another person where face-to-face interaction between carer and cared-for is a crucial element of the overall activity and where the need is of such a nature that it cannot possibly be met by the person in need herself' (Bubeck 1995: 129). She intends her definition to capture 'the more active and face-to-face aspects of care' including activities such as feeding, washing, lifting, and cleaning up the incontinent. Given our focus on the daily body work associated with home care, Bubeck's definition captures key elements of our conceptualisation of body work: face-to-face interactions, the relationality of care and the provision of care to those who cannot perform those activities themselves.

   In our analysis of this type of labour we address what Carol Wolkowitz (2006: 147) describes as 'employment that takes the body as its immediate site of labour, involving intimate, messy contact with the (frequently supine or naked) body, its orifices or products through close proximity'. In this category of body work the focus is on the physicality of bodies. Michael Fine (2007: 171) argues that 'recognition of the body and the precarious vulnerability of physical life provide a powerful conceptual tool with which to explore the central place that issues of care occupy in human societies'. However, the body's physical vulnerability also needs to be understood within a conceptual framing which recognises the creative capacity of the human subject; as Grosz (1994: xi) has argued, 'bodies are not inert, they function interactively and productively. They act and react'.

   In intimate body work the caregiver's body is the direct apparatus of care (Twigg 2002). In recognising the interaction of bodies (of caregivers and care recipients) in the production of lived experience, we are able to observe processes whereby powerful discourses concerning care are embodied in day-to-day encounters, such as those involved in home care. We find the lens of embodiment useful to our analysis: thinking about care from an embodied perspective, focuses on the experiential lived body (Twigg 2000, 2002, Wolkowitz 2006). For instance, in her study of the 'dirty work' of dealing with excrement in a mental hospital, van Dongen (2001: 205) notes nurses' 'disgust and contempt in relation to body wastes and care'. The affect (in this case, negative emotions) and power-laden relationship of care become particularly intense around the 'leaky body'. Although experiencing disgust, van Dongen found that nurses, drawing on their professionalism, do not blame patients and 'believe that even when cleaning, social, intimate contact is necessary' (2001: 209). In the hierarchy of jobs within the hospital, those doing this close, dirty work carry lower status.

Of interest here is van Dongen's analysis of the 'open' body (that leaks and 'fails') as placed appropriately in the hospital or the home, the latter representing private space where orifices and their leaking are a 'matter of care and intimacy' (2001: 208).

The hierarchies in the organisation of intimate body work, its commodification in formal care provision systems and the overlapping of, or empirical distinction between, 'caring for' (task-oriented, physical labour) and 'caring about' (relational, therapeutic emotional labour) all come together in the complex material and discursive fields making up the contemporary landscape of home care (Tronto 1993, Grant et al. 2004, Theodosius 2008).[2] The site of the home blurs the conceptual distinction between 'caring for' and 'caring about', and Yeates (2004: 371) notes that the former refers to the performance or supervision of tasks, whereas the latter points up the 'perspectives and orientations, often integrated with tasks', and might include, for example, listening to someone's troubles and comforting them. At the same time, processes and policies associated with the neoliberal climate within which care is constructed reach deep into the actual practices of body work and the social practices of caregiving (Twigg 2002). In the rest of the chapter we turn to these practices, first briefly discussing the contextualisation of the study in the national and regional framing of home care practice, its methods and data.

The study and its context

Home care in Canada is not covered by the federal Canada Health Act that regulates the provincial and territorial health insurance programs. Instead the provinces and territories determine the contours of formal home care provision in their jurisdiction, leading to variation across the country regarding eligibility and the extent and nature of home care provision (Coyte and McKeever 2001, Armstrong and Armstrong 2003). Ontario used to deliver home care primarily through the public sector, but in the mid-1990s introduced new public management techniques. Home care was restructured around a process of competitive bidding for contracts from service providers in the non-profit and the for-profit sectors. This was later accompanied by restricting eligibility, delisting some services and rationing hours of publicly funded home provision (England et al. 2007).

The restructuring of home care occurred within broader healthcare reform involving hospital closures, and releasing patients sooner to save money. Shorter hospital stays and faster discharges reveal cultural assumptions about home and a strong normative expectation that a network of family and friends is able and willing to step in to provide care at home. Shifting financial responsibility for care onto individuals may be potentially cost-saving from the perspective of the province, but the families often end up paying for supplies and services that would be included if the same care was in a hospital or nursing home. Home care reform has meant more and different work for workers and increasing the workload of family caregivers (Aronson and Neysmith 1997, England et al. 2007).

Our analysis draws from an ethnographic study and quantitative survey of clients from across Ontario who had received publicly funded long-term care services. The project explored different dimensions of this landscape of care. The ethnographic research dealt with 17 home care recipients and their paid care workers and family caregiver (if they had one). The clients, family caregivers and paid care workers were interviewed separately and were asked about various aspects of their experiences with long-term care provision. The material arrangements of homespace were described and photographed. All the care recipients in the study were clients of service providers contracted by one of three Community Care Access Centers (CCACs) across Ontario. The paid care workers were allocated by organisations that won contracts paid for by the province via the CCACs. Data from the study as a whole inform the themes discussed, but we focus here on the cases of Glenda, Sarah and Robert, whose care arrangements are particularly useful in tracing divisions of labour in body work and exploring how social policy plays out within dominant discourses of 'family' and paid labour. We draw on data from interviews with the three clients, four interviews with family caregivers and seven interviews with paid care workers (nurses, personal support workers and attendants).

Glenda, aged 82, is housebound and suffers from diabetes and arthritis, but is dying from lung cancer. She needs an oxygen tube and carries the oxygen tank on a pulley. Glenda lives with her daughter, Donna, and her son-in-law, Ben. Her daughter is listed as Glenda's primary caregiver, but Donna is also ill (with cancer) and is frequently bed-bound. So in practice, Glenda's son-in-law (who works full time as a teacher) provides most of the care, not only for his mother-in-law, but also for his wife when she is less well. A neighbour is also involved in Glenda's care arrangements. Sarah is aged 50 and has had Multiple Sclerosis (MS) for about 13 years and, while she needs a wheelchair, she is not housebound. She lives with her husband, Andy. Her paid care workers include Celia, a Personal Support Worker, Registered Practical Nurse Sandy, and Alexa, who is an attendant. The homemaker Celia is scheduled to work one hour each weekday with Sarah, but sometimes other workers do the shifts. Sandy, the RPN, visits Sarah approximately every third week (primarily for catherisation and assessment), and Alexa, the attendant goes in three times a week (other attendants go in the other days). Robert is 69 years old and he was diagnosed with MS about six years earlier. His wife, Diane, cares for him, and the paid care workers include PSW, Maggie, and Gina, an attendant. Maggie is there two evenings a week, and every other weekend evening for an hour. Gina visits Robert five mornings a week for 1.5 hours, two weekday afternoons for 30 minutes and a morning every other weekend.

Constituting care: body work as social and material practice

The data provided by the clients, workers and family caregivers in the three cases demonstrate the complexity of constituting care, a process that emerges from an interweaving not only of discursive understandings of family, homes and bodies, but also of policy and professional practice guidelines. Care is constituted through the interactions between particular bodies in the carrying out of care and, following Bubeck, the less tangible human dimension of care – one imbued with therapeutic emotional interpersonal labour. In home care, the client's home is both a workplace and private domestic space which in turn sets particular conditions under which care is provided. We consider this care space and then go on to themes emerging in the data that pertain to the negotiation and organisation of specific practices of body work.

The home is a workplace and domestic space
While the increased use of home care fits into the neoliberal frame of cost-containment and shorter hospital stays, it is also embedded in a discourse of being the preferred option, reiterated by care workers and family members. Nurses have long advocated more home-based rather than intuitional long-term care. Their work keeps people in their homes for as long as possible. Sandy (Sarah's RPN) commented, 'I think it's just so great to be able to go and see people at home and they're in their own environment and it's comfortable for them and it's great'. And Shirley (Glenda's RN) remarked 'elderly people that I've been seeing for years and years, they see you as the person that's trying to keep them at home.

You're the one who's really trying to not have them go to a nursing home'. The clients and family caregivers also valued home-based care, indicating gratitude that this was possible. Donna, for example, facing the impending death of her mother said:

> We're quite aware of what the future will bring. Ahm, me, but I think she does too. We both know. I'm very, VERY thankful that we have had this time. Thanks to the system, we have gained time that we would never have had and I'm very fortunate.

In contrast with institutional sites, the home as a site of care is a private space, embedded with personal and symbolic meanings. It is this dimension of home care that illuminates the distinction of the body as an object of care and the body as self or social being. The conceptual distinction between 'caring for' (task-oriented physical labour) and 'caring about' (relational, therapeutic emotional labour) reminds us that care work that is 'caring about' is not readily commodified, in contrast to the more measurable tasks of 'caring for' (Grant *et al.* 2004). Yet, empirically, in the case of body work in the home, we might anticipate, as Wolkowitz (2006) comments, an overlapping of the two and variations in how they are combined. When body work occurs in the personalised spatial context of the home, it becomes more difficult to reduce the client to a mere physical entity. The care workers and the clients are, of course, brought together because of the client's need for body work. While, from a social policy perspective, this might merely be a work relation based on 'caring for' the client's body, in practice it is often one that is infused with emotional labour that inflects the care relationship. When asked to describe her relationship with Glenda, for instance, Laurie (Personal Support Worker) replied 'She's just like a grandmother to me. I can laugh with her, I can joke with her, I can cry with her'. Sometimes care workers linked the 'caring about' aspect of their job to the home as a workplace:

> I do prefer it, though, because it is more personal, you get to know people but I mean you're not buddy-buddy, but you do, you have more time to talk, and you can work more according to their needs and respect (them) (Alexa, Sarah's Attendant).

The therapeutic emotional dimension of care transfers into how tasks are enacted. Maggie (Robert's PSW) captures this as she describes the sort of work she does:

> Each person has their own little thing that they want done. It could be something special like rubbing their back or making sure their feet are elevated enough that the heels don't rub on the sheet. Ahm, making sure that they have pads underneath them in case they are incontinent.

In Robert's case, Maggie has noticed and responded to his discomfort around wrinkled sheets. She visits him in the evenings to get him ready for bed.

> I make him feel comfortable. If there's the least little wrinkle under him, he'll let me know. And so you go back and fix whatever the problem is because you don't want somebody to be uncomfortable (Maggie, Robert's PSW).

Homes, however, are not designed for home care, and care workers encounter a wide variety of homes. Shirley (Glenda's Registered Nurse), for example, estimated that she has about

30 clients, so in effect she has 30 different workplaces. Across all the cases in the project, conditions varied from small, cluttered urban apartments to large suburban or rural single-family dwellings. Glenda, Sarah and Robert all live in single-family homes, Glenda and Robert's in rural villages and Sarah's in a suburb. Sarah and Robert's homes have been modified to accommodate wheelchair use and all three provide good working conditions for the care workers. The bedrooms and bathrooms of the clients are the most common spaces for providing intimate physical care of the body, the open, 'leaky' body – touching, lifting, undressing, giving enemas, changing catheters. Thus, this work transgresses the boundaries of 'normal' social interactions both in relation to bodily boundaries and in the use of 'private' homespaces. Respect, individuality, being mindful of their client's privacy (within their home, but also at the scale of the body) and treating their clients with dignity were common themes in interviews. Sensitivity to 'invasion' of the home was talked about by several workers, who elaborated on how they tried to mitigate this:

> When I first started this job our case manager was very ahm, strict and she made it very clear [. . .] we were to consider ourselves like a guest in their home and that we had to respect what they wanted done; and if there were things–like if they really didn't want a bath, if they didn't want certain things that we had to respect that (Shirley, RN for Glenda).

Nevertheless, the shift of homespace also to act as a workplace does have an impact on family caregivers' use of their own homes. Ben (Glenda's son-in-law) remarked, 'I'm rarely here when they are. I just try to keep out of their way'. He accepts that at least for the time the care workers are in his home, it is transformed into a paid workplace. Parts of the home might be changed because of equipment in the home (patient hoist devices are a case in point) or a stream of care workers coming through the house over the course of a day. Robert's bedroom is on the ground floor and his wife, Diane, lamented that in the evenings 'the living room is no good to me now'. She moved the TV upstairs to her bedroom, because the paid care workers' visits were an interruption. 'Yeah, that's what's gone for me, is my privacy in my house. And there's people coming and going pretty well all day long'. Household routines may also be adjusted to accommodate the care workers. Diane changed her morning routine: 'I don't want to interfere with the worker 'cause she's only got so much time and I don't want her having to wait while I get out of the bathroom'. In Glenda's case, Donna (daughter) makes sure she is available if a worker needs to speak to her. She and Shirley (RN) spend a good deal of time reviewing Glenda's condition and her medications to make sure the balance is right. Shirley commented:

> When I go in I usually check (Glenda's) vital signs, listen to her lungs, her blood sugars, see if she has had bladder infections. Usually I talk to Donna about the oxygen. I'm finding I'm having to check with Donna about more things because I don't find that Glenda's, ah, cognitive function is quite as good as it used to be.

Both family caregiver and paid care worker have similar goals in terms of the care of the care recipient, but their own experience of the same material space is tempered by the tension emerging as the meaning of home is re-worked when it is also enacted as a paid workplace. In addition, as we address in the next sections, the practices of body work are shaped by a complex interweaving of the regulatory mechanisms surrounding the provision of home care along with the physical and affective dimensions of intimate body work.

Regulating the body work of home care

Actual body work practices in the home reflect the reach of policy directives and the com-modification of care. Competitive bidding for home care contracts bears the stamp of managerialism, with its emphasis on quantification and economic rationality. Yet in prac-tice this emphasis and the difficulties in applying directives and their consequences are negotiated and may be resisted in bodily interactions of care workers and clients. Not all workers, however, have equal authority in such situations.

An important aspect of the commodification of care is that of time. As a way to save money and move workers more quickly through homes, agencies began quantifying par-ticular tasks by allocating them specific amounts of time. Shirley (Glenda's RN) described how she had her five minutes for a general assessment, 15 minutes to pour a week's worth of medicines, and so on. She noted that 'if my visits were too long, I would be told that I'm spending too long with the patients, [I'm told] what the acceptable amount of time is'. Nurses expressed general frustration that previously they had more autonomy and could use their professional judgement about their clients' need for services. Clients noticed the shift; Sarah commented that care workers.

> don't have time. They're trying to stay within a schedule. You're allowed so much time, you know. They will stay if there is a problem or, you know, to finish off your little talk about something, but they are trying to work within a schedule.

Sarah hints at one of the problems of placing time limits on care tasks; this commodification is certainly significant in managing the 'caring for' dimension of care. However, unlike physical body work, therapeutic emotional work (caring about) is less amenable to quan-tification. The care workers were conscious of this empirical distinction and the importance of going beyond the strict categorisation in their work. Shirley (Glenda's RN), for example, noted the time needed to provide care that went beyond simply the physical care of Glenda. After describing the tasks she carried out, she concluded: 'basically that's it, and I try to, you know, spend some time with her if there are things that she wants to talk to me about or if there's things that are kind of worrying her'. Shirley remarked that initially she was only allocated 30 minutes to see Glenda, and asked for more time:

> She's a palliative but she hadn't been coded that. So I coded her for emotional support, family support, I think I've got it up to 45 to 50 minutes. . . . (Glenda) felt the need to cry, she felt depressed about the fact she knows she's dying and that she feels she has to be very brave and not cry in front of Donna (Glenda's daughter), she's just trying to, you know, put up this, very stoic front. I just felt like how can I deal with this woman, give her any kind of comfort, and expect to do it in 30 minutes?

Personal Support Workers do not have the same power to recode or extend the time they are allocated to care for a client. It can be a struggle to fit everything into the time and there may be legal consequences of working beyond that allocated time. Celia (Sarah's PSW) described a recent experience with another client:

> She has a catheter and I was supposed to be in there for an hour to give her a bed bath, get her up in the Hoyer and get her into the living-room. Ah, it took an hour and a half because she'd had a BM [bowel movement] and she was mess from one end to the other and I had to clean it all up and ah, so it took longer. And we're supposed

to inform our company if we're spending any time more than necessary at a client's house because then we're not insured with Worker's Compensation.

Celia's comment indicates that some of the agencies' rules are informed by provincial regulations (in her case eligibility for medical care if she is injured on the job). Other agency rules govern which group of paid care workers can undertake what tasks. Gina and Maggie, Robert's attendant and personal support worker, gave examples of the minutiae of these regulations:

> We're not, ah, able to put cream on an open [wound] or anything like that. If you're washing somebody and they would like you to make sure that [the wound] is covered and cream put on, you know, things like that. If it's not open we can apply cream, but if it's open we can't. They have to have a registered nurse [. . .] applying the creams to any open areas (Gina, Robert's attendant).

> We're not allowed to take the medications out of the bottle and hand them to them. [. . .] that's family or themselves or an RN that's classified to do that. I can hand them the bottle, I open the bottle, but I can't take the pills out of the bottle (Maggie, Robert's PSW).

These comments reflect how agencies' rules produce and reinforce a division of labour among the home care workers, as well as one between paid workers and family caregivers (discussed in the next section) and also highlight the potential negotiation of care that may emerge between care workers and clients. This was of particular concern when there were changes of care workers. How the agencies schedule workers can mean multiple carers and discontinuities of care, which potentially has more impact in home care than it would in a hospital or nursing home. The anxiety is around potential disruptions – particularly in terms of knowledge, whether this is knowledge about routine needs or the specifics about carrying out particular practices. For example, Diane (Robert's wife) was concerned because one of the paid care workers was to have surgery and would be replaced temporarily:

> It's somebody new and you'll have to go through where everything is and, you know, it's a [. . .] sensitive thing, someone in your house every day. I think that the (agencies) feel that shouldn't matter, just as long as you get somebody. But I think they are leaning maybe toward having a little more feeling for us, seeing it our way. I think the workers find it better too, if they're here on a regular basis.

Diane and Sarah both expressed exasperation that they repeatedly had to explain the particularities of their situations because of the turnover in paid care workers or temporary replacements. Diane emphasised that Robert needed routine and consistency in his daily regime: 'he likes things on schedule and it's upsetting to him, even the little details, like he wants his coffee before he shaves' and she relies on the care workers to help her provide that structured framework for Robert. For Diane, the turnover of workers, or more critically, when they do not turn up, causes her stress. She frames their role in Robert's care in terms of expertise. She admits she can do some of the tasks, but feels 'he doesn't get the good care, you know. I can't do all the little details like they would. I have to just cut corners and do what I'm able to do'.

For Sarah, lack of continuity could have a profound effect on her care. Her narrative, in particular, demonstrated her active agency in the management of gaps in the system.

Sarah requires considerable intimate body work, and she is sometimes compelled to take control of this body work. She recounts the distressing experience of a new RPN who had problems inserting the urinary catheter. Sarah's view was that the RPN was inexperienced, but later discovered that the RPN had written in her chart that multiple catheters were used because Sarah could not keep her legs open. This was not the case, so she asked that a different RPN be sent. She also devised a technique using a long sock to make catheterisations easier for the paid care worker and more comfortable for her, and proceeded to teach it to each care worker. Care is often presented as one-directional, something that is performed on a passive recipient. However, Sarah's case shows that experiential knowledge of body work is transmitted back to paid care workers. Her RPN, Sandy, commented that Sarah is 'very knowledgeable about her disease [. . .] she's also very realistic about it' which made Sandy's job easier. Sandy talked about Sarah giving her instructions about the 'tricks' that work for her: 'she just tells you how to do it and yeah, so I mean that isn't a problem'. Sarah had not always been so assertive. She had fallen from a patient hoist device twice before, and spoke frequently of being nervous about people lifting and moving her. Since the second fall she had decided to be more direct with the workers, 'you feel vulnerable,' she said, 'it's your body that's going down on the floor, you know'.

In practice, to complete the body work for Glenda, Sarah and Robert requires a fine balance and that balance is often fragile. Oftentimes this fragility is revealed in the lack of continuity of care. It may also be because of a lack of care – the interview data included examples of care workers getting sick or snowed in and there was no-one available to replace them. This may well be an issue that is more problematic when care is carried out in the home rather than a hospital setting. Added to this is the need for family caregivers to attend to their own self-care, as they are a constant link in the chain of care, they are, as Diane (Robert's wife) put it, 'the back-up, the contingency plan'. In the next section we consider the divisions of labour in care that underpin the provision of care – both in terms of 'caring for' and 'caring about'.

Divisions of labour in body work
When body care is provided by a combination of family caregivers and paid care workers, primary responsibility for specific tasks is usually assigned to particular people. These divisions of body work reflect not only professional practice hierarchies, but also a working out among family members, paid workers and care recipients, about who has responsibility for which care tasks. Our interview data indicate that divisions of labour (between family caregivers and paid care workers) in a particular home can become routinised, especially once all concerned have established relationships.

The occupational hierarchy within paid home care work in the community usually reflects the amount of education and training received, pay levels and prestige, and the specific tasks associated with each occupation. RNs are increasingly associated with the more technical, administrative and informational aspects of care, especially as they move up the ranks – and away from close bodily involvement. They are distanced from the 'dirty work' of actual intimate body work (Twigg 2000) and are more likely to do assessments and more technical care tasks. The personal support workers and attendants do more of the labour-intensive activities and the 'dirty work' associated with the close bodily care of others. How family caregivers are involved is less prescribed, and in the three cases considered here they participate in body work on the client in different ways and to varying extents.

Sarah actively created a division of body work that excluded her husband, Andy. She valued and made use of the gradations of difference between worker, friend and family member as care provider:

I prefer to have Andy's help as a caregiver as little as possible, simply because if your husband becomes your caregiver, then he isn't your husband any more. The relationship is blurred there. If I still want to be a person unto myself, then I don't want to include him in some parts of care, like a bowel treatment or a shower day.

Andy, her husband, mirrored this when he described, a little awkwardly, his care responsibilities as 'I guess mental companion, you know, someone to talk to. If necessary, physical care, ah, you know, getting her into her chair, getting her into the bed. Those would probably be it'. Sarah is very clear about her identity as a wife as well as her wish not to be reduced to be the object of body work.

Glenda's care could be described as a mixed economy: she has formal care, informal care from her family, and private paid care. There was a clear division of duties between Ben (son-in-law) and Donna (daughter), as well as between them and the paid workers. For instance, Glenda's twice daily insulin injections are given by Ben because of his knowledge and expertise. Donna said 'we were both shown in the hospital how to do the needle. One of us paid attention, and that would be him'. Similarly, Ben is also in charge of the strong medicines because he 'has a chemistry background'. However, Ben and the workers were all clear that Donna makes the decisions about Glenda's care and she manages the division of responsibilities. Certain tasks fell directly in the mandate of the attendants: 'They give her her bath. They don't clean her room. They feed her, they prepare food, I think that's the main thing, and they take care of her bed' (Donna).

In addition to the two publicly funded paid care workers, Shirley (RN) and Laurie (PSW), Donna hired their neighbour, Irene, to help clean the house and provide additional personal care for Glenda not covered by the system. At a minimum, Irene is in their home twice a week, but she also drives Donna and Glenda to their medical appointments and to get their groceries. Irene is clearly a very important node in Glenda's care; she was mentioned very warmly by all three members of the family, and even the PSW. Glenda enthused 'I'll always keep Irene; she's part of our family. Irene's like a piece of furniture here, she's well liked, she's become part of the household'. Beyond demonstrating that sometimes extra care is bought privately, Glenda's situation shows how finely balanced care arrangements are. Glenda, Donna, Ben and the PSW each talked about an overnight trip Ben took to attend a conference and the complicated arrangements put in place to give Glenda insulin. In turn, Ben finds caring for 'the ladies', as he calls them, as well as working full time, very demanding:

> I think one of the things that bothers me is that I have to be at a certain place at a certain time. Mum needs her injections twice a day, Donna doesn't like to do it, she needs her medications, she needs her meals pretty much on time, and proper balanced diet. [. . .] So it's just ah, from morning to night it's rush, rush, rush, get this done, get that done. I'm just bone weary.

In Robert's case, Diane depends on the workers because much of Robert's care involves lifting and moving him and she is physically unable to do that because of back problems. She makes sure that he has opportunities to socialise with his friends; she is strict about getting him to do his exercises and swimming weekly to keep his body supple so he can be moved more easily. Diane has told the agency she does not want the assistance offered with cooking his meals. She and Robert prefer that she makes his meals. In this way she is providing him with some sense of domestic normalcy and continuity of their long-established domestic arrangements. However, the most intimate personal care, like a daily bowel movement and showering, is usually undertaken by PSW Maggie or attendant Gina.

> (Robert) needs a bowel routine every morning, so I give him a suppository. And then he just stays in bed until he feels that it's going to work. [. . .] So he has his bowel movement and then ah, I give him a shower and then dress him (Gina, Robert's attendant).

Of course, that it is the attendant and PSW providing these most bodily of personal care activities reflects broader occupational divisions. These aspects of body work are tasks least likely to be undertaken by family members. Delegating these tasks to non-family members can be seen as a means of maintaining the clients' dignity within their families. Diane, however, is still involved in such care from time to time:

> Sometimes he'll have a bowel accident in the chair so I try to clean that up, and ah . . . they might send somebody in for that, but I think by the time they could find someone it might be quite a while that he had to sit in it, so we do manage it.

The divisions of labour around the 'dirty work' of home care were striking. Diane will deal with Robert's excrement if need be, Sarah is extremely reluctant to have her husband involved in that aspect of her care. Shirley (RN) and Sandy (RPN) did not do much of the body work associated with body wastes. They did catherisations and checked blood levels, but cleaning up body waste and bowel routines were not part of their official duties (this is also the general trend across the other cases in the larger project). Reflecting Twigg's (2002) observations about hierarchies in nursing, in home care the work of RNs and even of many RPNs is 'marked by distance from the body and direct body work' (Twigg 2002: 428). The 'dirty work' was more squarely the task of PSWs and attendants like Maggie and Gina.

Discussion

In their anthology on care work, Zimmerman *et al.* (2006: 3–4) explain that they

> deliberately chose the term 'care work' to refer to the multifaceted labour that produces the daily living conditions that make basic human health and well-being possible. [. . .] (and) because it acknowledges these multiple facets, especially the important emotional dimensions involved (*i.e.* care), coupled with the complexity and physical demands (*i.e.* work).

While a useful definition as far as it goes, in this chapter we have presented a more nuanced understanding of care work by focusing on the body, the care worker–client relationship and the home as a site of care work. The home in various ways shapes how care is provided and how all the parties involved experience homespace. The materiality and meanings of home provide conditions under which regarding the body as simply a physical object is hard to sustain. Caring for this body almost inevitably involves the forming of relationships between family caregivers, care workers and care recipients that are predicated on the interweaving of the materiality of the body to be 'cared for' and a sense of a self to be 'cared about' that subverts a reading of the body solely in terms of its physical care needs. The paid care worker/care recipient relationship is further informed by a desire to distance bodily needs from a valued identity on the part of the client, and their wish to engage in 'normal' social interactions.

Close bodily interactions associated with personal care are central to activities and experiences associated with home. When home care workers and family caregivers together engage in the intimate care of the bodies of clients, however, these bodily interactions are interpreted and enacted within a wider context of meanings about bodies and homespace. The home, as a material and symbolic space is imbued with a legacy of powerful notions of family, privacy and control. Home care workers transgress 'appropriate' personal boundaries, and also enter the most intimate spaces of the home (bedrooms and bathrooms) in the course of body work; consequently, established meanings of bodies and homespace need to be renegotiated (Dyck et al. 2005). Care work remains deeply gendered, and implicit in home care reform. Men, however, like Andy and Ben in this study, are increasingly involved in providing care to family members, raising new questions about how care work, often under valued and rarely recognised as a learnt skill and hard work, is accommodated in gender identities (Folbre and Nelson 2000).

Policy directives which commodify care also operate in particular ways to inform how care is put into practice and how specific decisions are rationalised. Furthermore, the organisation of paid care, particularly with respect to gaps in continuity of care, has effects on how the embodied knowledge of care recipients themselves may become a crucial part of their care (as in the case of Sarah's instructions to care workers). While the divisions of labour between paid and family caregivers may seem clear-cut, our analysis reveals how coordination is an important aspect of ensuring good care for the recipient. A fine balance of the divisions of labour, sometimes fragile, is achieved as paid and family caregivers and care recipients come together in managing the body work in the specific space of a home that doubles as a workplace. This includes families reorganising their time and even their homespace to cope with their home as someone else's workplace. There can be problems with home care, but all the clients and their family caregivers indicated gratitude for home care. Despite the stress in the families, it was highly valued, especially as a means of keeping their families together at home despite profound illnesses.

As Michael Fine (2007: 178) points out 'the body in care is considerably more complex than a focus on the body of the care recipient alone might indicate'. The experiences of Glenda, Sarah, Robert, their families and paid care workers offer 'lived body' evidence supporting Fine's claim. The relationship between care recipient and care worker is often an emotionally complex and deeply power-inflected one, and unlike work relations in an institution, the home-based care work relation has a greater potential to be shaped by intimacy, affective labour and ideologies of friendship and family. Using the case of publicly funded home care, we argue that body work should be repositioned, and analyses need to include the embodied knowledge of both those providing and receiving care. In foregrounding this knowledge, body work can be understood as actively co-constituted by caregivers and care recipients through negotiation of micro-practices in the home; practices which, however, are shaped by regulatory mechanisms beyond the home which interweave in complex ways with the affective dimensions of care and its intimacy. Drawing on, and extending the concept of body work to analyse the dynamics of long-term care relations and practices in private homes provides new ways of understanding both the material and non-material relations and processes of the shifting care landscape that shapes the lives of some of the most vulnerable of our populations.

Acknowledgements

We thank the clients, their families and the care workers for their time, energy and enthusiasm in participating in this research. The interviews we draw on were conducted by Pia Kontos, and additional research assistance was provided by Caitlin Henry. We are grateful to both of them. Finally we greatly appreciate the guidance of the editors of the book in helping us produce a stronger chapter.

Notes

1   The names of the clients, family caregivers and care workers are pseudonyms. The empirical research for this chapter is part of a larger project on home care in Ontario funded by the Social Sciences and Humanities Research Council of Canada. The research team was led by Principal Investigator Patricia McKeever, and includes Co-Investigators: J. Angus, M. Chipman, A. Dolan, I. Dyck, J. Eakin, K. England, D. Gastaldo, B. Poland, and Research Co-ordinator K. Osterlund.
2   Our ideas about emotional labour are informed by the ongoing lively debates about theorising emotion and identifying different sorts of emotional labour. Here we use emotional labour to mean the interactive (even collaborative) relational and reflective aspects of care work. We draw on Catherine Theodosius's (2008: 146) notion of therapeutic emotional labour as the sort of emotional labour where 'the nurse's intention is to enable the establishment or maintenance of the interpersonal therapeutic relationship between nurse and patient in a way that facilitates their movement towards independent healthy living'. Also helpful is Liz Bondi's (2008) conceptualisation of care work as a paradoxical, emotionally laden interpersonal relationship. Our use of 'caring about' also reflects, to some extent, the 'caring about' phase of Joan Tronto's (1993) four ethical dimensions of care: being aware of and attentive to care needs and well-being of others.

References

Armstrong, P. and Armstrong, H. (2003) *Wasting Away: the Undermining of Canadian Healthcare*, 2nd Edition. Toronto: Oxford University Press.
Aronson, J. and Neysmith, S.M. (1997) The retreat of the state and long-term care provision: implications for frail elderly people, unpaid family carers and paid home care workers, *Studies in Political Economy*, 53, 37–65.
Bondi, L. (2008) On the relational dynamics of caring: a psychotherapeutic approach to emotional and power dimensions of women's care work, *Gender, Place and Culture*, 15, 3, 249–65.
Bubeck, D. (1995) *Care, Gender and Justice*. Oxford: Clarendon Press.
Coyte, P.C. and McKeever, P. (2001) Home care in Canada: passing the buck, *Canadian Journal of Nursing Research*, 33, 2, 11–25.
Dyck, I., Kontos, P., Angus, J. and McKeever, P. (2005) The home as a site for long-term care: meanings and management of bodies and spaces, *Health and Place*, 11, 173–85.
England, K., Eakin, J., Gastaldo, D. and McKeever, P. (2007) Neoliberalizing home care: managed competition and restructuring home care in Ontario. In England, K. and Ward, K. (eds) *Neoliberalization: Networks, States, Peoples*. Oxford: Blackwell.
Fine, M. (2007) *A Caring Society?: Care and the Dilemmas of Human Service in the Twenty-first Century*. New York: Palgrave-Macmillan.
Folbre, N. and Nelson, J.A. (2000) For love or money – or both? *Journal of Economic Perspectives*, 14, 4, 123–40.
Grant, K., Amaratunga, C., Armstrong, P., Boscoe, M., Pederson, A. and Willson, K. (eds) (2004) *Caring For/Caring About: Women, Home Care, and Unpaid Caregiving*. Aurora, Ont: Garamond Press.

Grosz, E. (1994) *Volatile Bodies. Toward a Corporeal Feminism*. Bloomington: Indiana University Press.

Held, V. (2006) *The Ethics of Care: Personal, Political, and Global*. Oxford: Oxford University Press.

Kittay, E.F. (1999) *Love's Labor: Essays on Women, Equality and Dependency*. New York: Routledge.

Sevenhuijsen, S. (1998) *Citizenship and the Ethics of Care: Feminist Considerations on Justice, Morality and Politics*. New York: Routledge.

Theodosius, C. (2008) *Emotional Labour in Health Care: the Unmanaged Heart of Nursing*. London: Routledge.

Tronto, J. (1993) *Moral Boundaries: a Political Argument for an Ethic of Care*. New York: Routledge.

Twigg, J. (2000) *Bathing, the Body and Community Care*. London: Routledge.

Twigg, J. (2002) The body in social policy: mapping a territory, *Journal of Social Policy*, 31, 3, 421–40.

van Dongen, E. (2001) It isn't something to yodel about, but it exists! Faeces, nurses, social relations and status within a mental hospital, *Aging and Mental Health*, 5, 3, 205–15.

Wolkowitz, C. (2006) *Bodies at Work*. Thousand Oaks, CA: Sage.

Yeates, N. (2004) Global care chains: critical reflections and lines of enquiry, *International Feminist Journal of Politics*, 6, 3, 369–91.

Zimmerman, M.K., Litt, J.S. and Bose, C.E. (2006) *Global Dimensions of Gender and Carework*. Stanford: Stanford University Press.

4

The means of correct training: embodied regulation in training for body work among mothers
Emma Wainwright, Elodie Marandet and Sadaf Rizvi

Introduction

Within the context of the UK Government's neo-liberal efforts to combat social exclusion by encouraging a shift from welfare to work through a strategy of (re)training, this chapter draws on research that explores some of the types of training courses being taken by mothers. More specifically, it explores the experiences of mothers taking training for body work or 'body training' in the areas of health, beauty and social care, (Wainwright *et al.* 2010) linked, in part, to notable skills gaps in the local West London economy where research was conducted.

The focus of this chapter is specifically on mothers' learning experiences, as 'non-working'[1] parents and in particular, mothers, have become a politically visible and high profile group in the UK (McDowell *et al.* 2005a,b). For example, the Skills for Life agenda (DfEE 2001) defines this group as its sixth most important in terms of literacy, language and numeracy targets (Appleby and Bathmaker 2006). But the prominence of parents – and especially mothers – is best evidenced through the high profile New Deal for Lone Parents (see Smith *et al.* 2008) which 'encourages' a return to work for mothers through the intermediary of (re)training. As discussed in relation to previous research (Wainwright *et al.* in press a), (re)training is considered a 'respectable' location (Skeggs 1997) especially among migrants, lone parents and those not in paid employment, pointing to efforts to make a transition to the workplace, financial independence and security.

Both theoretically and empirically, the processes of training and training spaces have been largely absent in the now numerous appraisals of various employment areas defined as body work (though see Gale 2007 for a detailed exception). But within an increasingly neo-liberalised socio-economic policy climate, training processes and spaces, along with the experiences of those undertaking training, warrant further exploration (see Smith *et al.* 2008). Moreover, very little has been written on the recursive relationship between training spaces and experiences of learning the necessary bodily and emotional skills for these types of work and the subsequent transferral to the workplace. Yet a focus on training enables much insight to be yielded into body work; on *how* the bodily is learned and enforced, not just its practice in the final workplace destination.

The role of the body in the workplace has become a fruitful area for sociological research over the past decade, with a recent flurry of more spatially nuanced approaches at a range

Body Work in Health and Social Care, First Edition. Edited by Julia Twigg, Carol Wolkowitz, Rachel Lara Cohen and Sarah Nettleton.
Chapters © 2011 The Authors. Book compilation © 2011 Foundation for the Sociology of Health & Illness / Blackwell Publishing Ltd. Published 2011 by Blackwell Publishing Ltd.

of scales (Dyer *et al.* 2008, McDowell 2009, Wainwright *et al.* in press b). This has gained particular impetus and credence with the growth of the service sector and its perceived 'feminisation' in terms of relevant skills, job opportunities and pervasive consumer culture, and the proliferation of work focusing on the 'improvement' of bodies, most especially female bodies (Gimlin 2007). Moreover, the 'rediscovery of the senses' in consumer culture has, according to Jutte (2005: 238, in Paterson 2007), validated 'new pleasure in the body', bringing together the embodied with the affective.

The research from which this chapter comes, together with previous research (Wainwright *et al.* 2010), has found that the choice of 'body training' courses that focus on the embodied, the emotional and, by extension, the care of others, are popular among mothers for various reasons linked to the expectation and performativity of a feminised and, very often, perceived 'natural' maternal identity, linking together home, family, work and leisure.[2] Though training choices are not the focus of this chapter, this indicates that gendered perceptions of skills and interests are still widely held by women, particularly mothers, and are perpetuated and reinforced by tutors, training advisors and governmental policy (Osgood 2005, Skeggs 1997). This chapter thus points to the pervasive and often implicit role of normative gender and maternal identity in the embodied regulation of training in 'caring' areas of body work and suggests that this stereotyping of women's and mothers' skills and training abilities is decidedly problematic.

By drawing on the notion of body work as both the interaction between bodies and the (self)disciplining of one's own body, this chapter discusses the varied regulatory processes of learning, from the embedding and embodying of 'professional' knowledge and identities, to the repressing of cultural norms and behaviour. With this focus on training and thinking through regulation, our main contention here is that the closer the work with the body the more urgent is the need for regulation of one's own body and the more fine-tuned the embodied discipline. We explore how this is often an implicitly gendered process with a tempering of certain constructed feminine performances and identities. Moreover, by focusing on a range of courses which fall under the rubric of interactional body work, we can see that mothers' varied experiences of training belie some important similarities which point to the pertinence of this body work framing.

The chapter begins by arguing that training spaces be seen as transitional and liminal – conceptual and physical spaces of 'in betweenness' – in which body work is taught and learnt for eventual practice in the workplace. The chapter then frames body work by detailing key literature and arguments. We then provide brief details on the 'body training' research project before tracing the training process through a set of embodied regulatory forms and their occasional subversion.

Liminal training spaces

We conceptualise training for body work as a physical and conceptual space of transition. For the cohort of students explored here, it is a space that sits at the nexus of public and private and home, work and leisure, and is where the individual moves from student to practitioner / worker requiring new and changing identities to be negotiated and regulated.

The concept of liminality encapsulates this very dynamism. For example, Shields (1991) employs it to express a transition from one life stage to another, and Pratt (2004) uses it to explain the experiences of and locations in which Filipina migrant women make transitions to family care work in Canada. Moreover, O'Conner and Madge (2005) draw on it to explore the use of parenting websites by women with new-born babies in transforming themselves into mothers.

Drawing on these varied uses of liminality, Buckingham *et al.* (2006) develop the concept to understand the sphere of training and to effectively describe how training spaces are variously inscribed by and for mothers. They suggest that mothers use training to perform different identities, try out different roles, and develop networks and portfolios, rather than using it merely as a transition to paid employment (also see Wainwright *et al.* in press a). Similarly, in our research here, the mothers we spoke to were motivated to take training for various reasons: as an extension of leisure interests, as a social activity, as a means of temporarily escaping their caring responsibilities, as well as to enable transition to the workplace.

Taking this argument forward and thinking through the specificities of our research, the training environment is made up of a range of different spaces and microgeographies through which transitions in identity and location are made. For example and at its most basic, while training primarily takes place in the classroom, it extends beyond to incorporate placements. Most students, especially in the care courses discussed here, are required to gain work experience in a 'real' care setting, working and interacting with 'real' patients / children and so forth. But also the quasi-public realm of the health and beauty courses requires the classroom to be transformed into a working salon with visiting clients. In this case, the training space changes in very material ways – from a more typical site of learning, with desks, chairs, white board, textbooks and tutor – to a site for practising body work, with benches, cubicles and clients. This is also a sensuous transformation with changes in lighting, sound and ambience aimed at creating a restorative experience for the 'client' (Wainwright *et al.* in press b).

Within this context, training is a site of and for various interactions: between tutor and students, among the students themselves, and in instances of practice, between students and their various 'client' groups. These spaces then involve a transition from learner to practitioner with a professional identity in the making. Training sits at the intersection of public and private, forming a bridge between the private space of home and the public space of economic encounter through paid employment.

Some writers such as Turner (1984: 44) have used liminality to explore spaces in which humans are 'liberated from the normative constraints of social structures'. While Buckingham *et al.* (2006) have similarly argued in relation to the multiple and complex uses of training by mothers, a focus on the actual training process shows that rather than liberation from normative constraints, these spaces are ones of close scrutiny where certain rules, regulations and performances are clearly etched out on and demanded of the body and its emotions. We highlight this now through our framings of the varied and interlinked conceptualisations of body work.

Framings

Interactional body work

The first conceptualisation of body work that we draw on is work that focuses on the interaction between bodies. Wolkowitz (2002) suggests that this incorporates 'many of the most important features of body work in contemporary society' (2002: 497) to include the varied experiences of those whose paid work involves the 'care, adornment, pleasure, discipline and cure' of others' bodies, stressing labour that involves intimate and often messy contact with the body through touch or close proximity. And this interpretation and conceptualisation of body work has been used to detail a varied number of employment types and spaces including studies of nursing (van Dongen and Elema 2001), professionalism and therapeutic massage (Oerton 2004), beauty therapy and the beauty salon (Sharma and Black 2001, Gimlin 1996) and home and the bodily dimensions of carework (Twigg 2000a, b, 2006).

But beyond a contained focus on the bodily and embodied of this work, much of this literature incorporates an emotional dimension that care of/for bodies frequently requires (Gimlin 2007). Twigg (2000a,b) and Milligan (2000, 2003) for example, have drawn attention to both the physicality and emotionality of caring, pointing to how care work is implicitly entangled in gendered meanings of home and identity (see also Evans and Thomas 2009). Further, Sharma and Black (2001), focusing on the emotional labour of beauty therapy, found that therapists defined their work in terms of work with feelings as well as with the body, stressing the importance of what it does to make women *feel* better. Thoroughly intertwined, the more intimate the contact and handling of bodies, the more necessary the sensitive handling of emotions.

Explicitly teasing out the emotional nature of embodiment (Davidson and Milligan 2004), Kang (2003) uses the term body labour to assign gendered work that involves management of emotions in body-related service provision. In using this term, she overtly conjoins the notion of body work with that of emotional labour as designated by Hochschild (1983). Emotional labour refers to the effort employers require workers to put into evoking or shaping, as well as suppressing, feelings in themselves and others. Using the detailed example of flight attendants, Hochschild (1983) argued that emotional labour requires face-to-face or voice-to-voice contact with customers or clients, that employees produce a certain emotional state in others, and methods of training and supervision give the employer control over workers' feelings (see Gimlin 2007: 361). Emotional labour therefore is about the emotions of the person who is the 'object' of the labour in question and the emotions of the person who performs the labour (Sharma and Black 2001).

As already flagged, resonating through conceptualisations and practices of body work and its emotional dimensions is the issue of gender; body work has been and continues to be primarily undertaken by women, and is based upon a sexual division of labour that assigns to women the care of bodies and the spaces they inhabit (Smith 1988):

> Whether it be in the field of basic nursing, massage, beauty therapy or sex work . . . contemporary sex/gender power relations tend to relegate the hands-on care of others' bodies, and the spaces they occupy, to women. (Oerton 2004: 561)

In many employment areas defined as body work, the actual corporeal process of handling and caring for bodies is commonly apportioned to those on the lower rungs or in the basic stages of the job (Oerton 2004, Twigg 2000a). This parallels women's continued horizontal and vertical segregation in paid employment that ascribe them to the lower echelons of traditionally female occupations. For example, in areas of body work that have been the focus of governmental drives to challenge existing gender segregation, such as childcare and nursing, men engaged in these are more likely to rise to more highly valued and responsible positions (Simpson 2004), thus moving away from embodied practices.

What is more, and of significance for our research here, is that body work has been further conceptualised through a maternalised discourse of care and familial responsibility: 'Because women do this work for babies and children, these activities are generalised as female' (Twigg 2000a: 407). Through essentialist and performed (self)constructions of women's abilities to mother, nurture, care and support (Brush 1999, Skeggs 1997, Wainwright *et al.* 2010), the notion of body work very often extends the geographies of mothers' care from the home to the world of paid employment.

Regulatory body work
The second meaning of body work we draw on here refers to the (self)disciplining which employees, particularly women, are expected to do on their own bodies. Although it has been shown that women learn to discipline their own bodies at a young age and well before they enter paid employment or start on their 'professional lives' (Young 1990), one key location for understanding this disciplining process has been the workplace. A highly gendered form of surveillance with regard to meeting and complying with the norms and expectations of the workplace, employers and organisational culture has been recognised (Halford *et al.* 1997, Shilling 1993, Williams 1998). Much of this work has taken a Foucauldian tack (Foucault 1977) to explore the disciplining function of the male gaze within the workplace (McDowell 1997, Tretheway 1999). It is this we want to reflect on here.

Though very widely drawn on across the social sciences, Foucault's *Discipline and Punish* (1977) is especially fruitful in an examination of the training process. In discussing the production of docile bodies and the processes by which we are made, the role of the body is central. Whether in considering the making of the ideal soldier in the 18th century where 'posture is gradually corrected; a calculated constraint runs slowly through each part of the body, mastering it, making it pliable, ready at all times . . .' (1977: 135) or the circulation of disciplinary techniques through various institutional bodies and geographies, Foucault impressively details how the Classical age discovered the body as both object and target of power. This is a body that is 'manipulated, shaped, trained, which obeys, responds, becomes skilful and increases its forces' (1977: 136) and the minutiae of this reveal how the individual is transformed, improved and made acceptable for the workplace.

Training for body work can be read as a set of corrections framed around the body of the student. In the direct words of Foucault (1977: 170), the aim is to train 'the moving, confused, useless multitude of bodies and forces into a multiplicity of individual elements – small, separate cells, organic autonomies, genetic identities and continuities, combinatory segments'. Thus 'the means of correct training' in a range of institutions and organisations was based on '. . . a whole micro-penality of time (lateness, absences, interruptions of tasks), of activity (inattention, negligence, lack of zeal), of behaviour (impoliteness, disobedience), of speech (idle chatter, insolence), of the body ('incorrect' attitudes, irregular gestures, lack of cleanliness), of sexuality (impurity, indecency)' (Foucault 1977: 178). Though this passage signals the materiality of the body as an important element of this disciplining work, Foucault's focus on the design of practices rather than how they actually worked means that it received little attention in his analysis. In this chapter we take some of these bodily dimensions of discipline – behaviour, speech, body and sexuality – to explore how their regulation is integral to the processes of training for body work, especially in relation to the regulation of the female body. And, moreover, how these take on greater urgency the closer in you get to the body and working with other bodies.

As Foucault did not dwell on gender, it has been left to the work of feminists to interrogate the ways women have accepted and subverted such embodied and often highly gendered disciplining. Within early workplace research, there was a clear undertaking to understand the ways in which women train their bodies to fit in with the prevailing organisational culture. For example, McDowell (1997) and McDowell and Court's (1994) focus on women employed in the City of London found that some of the women working in merchant banks felt obliged to tame their own bodies in ways deemed appropriate to

Table 1 *Subject areas researched*

Caring	Adorning	Curing	Pleasuring
Childcare	Nail technology	Reflexology	Massage
Carework	Hairdressing	Aromatherapy	
Nursing	Beauty therapy		
	Waxing		

operating in a masculinised environment, such as adopting a masculinist work dress and becoming honorary men (Acker 1990). Sometimes considered mundane forms of body work, consideration of various body management practices including washing, brushing teeth, hairstyling, and application of makeup have warranted increased attention (see Gimlin 2007 for an overview). The body training environment is especially useful for flagging how these seemingly trivial yet essential work codes are instilled through normalising and social conditioning.

The 'body training' project

This chapter is based on fieldwork undertaken as part of a project on the 'body-training choices, expectations and experiences of mothers in West London'[3]. As its starting point, this has loosely drawn on Wolkowitz's (2002 and 2006) aforementioned body work categories of caring, adorning, curing and pleasuring to examine a range of subject areas (see table 1)[4].

Though all linking to interactional body work, we recognise that the subject areas discussed here are very different. But we can usefully view them together – looking at their commonalities – to see the significance of the (self)disciplined body when encountering, in an often very intimate way, the bodies of others – whether children, patients or clients – in a caring capacity. In so doing we can explore, among other issues, how the embodied physicality and emotionality of body training in health, beauty and social care are learned, taught and negotiated.

As a qualitatively-based project, we draw here on approximately 30 interviews with the nine course tutors, two two-hour scoping focus groups with mothers taking the courses (designated as caring, adorning, curing and pleasuring) and two waves of one-to-one and paired-depth interviews with 32 enrolled mothers. These lasted from 30 minutes to one hour.

Courses to recruit from were chosen on the advice of tutors as being courses popular among mothers. The sample chosen was opportunistic and depended upon participant suitability, availability and willingness. Focus groups were used to elicit initial experiences relating to training and motherhood. Following these and using a semi-structured interview format, in-depth interviews with mothers were then conducted. The first interview took place towards the beginning of their course and the second close to the end (with approximately six months in between). These were used to gauge details of how the learning process is experienced and its link to maternal and gender identities. With permission, interviews and focus groups were audio-recorded and transcribed.

Though participants were familiar with the research team by the time of the interviews, paired-depth interviews – whereby participants were interviewed in twos – were offered as a 'safe space' in which to discuss issues and experiences (Pratt 2002). Led by feminist iological critiques of the research process, we sought to enable participation through, io ample, payment of incurred childcare costs and encouraged participant questioning of and involvement in the research and its outcomes.

The interviewed students varied in age from their early 20s to late 40s and, reflecting the West London area, were ethnically diverse. In presenting qualitative data here, we use numbers to identify different tutors and pseudonyms for those mothers with whom we conducted in-depth interviews. Due to identification problems, mothers in the focus groups are not separately named.

In the absence of access to data on the student body, we cannot say how far our interviewees are representative of all those taking body training courses. Instead, what we offer is insight into the regulatory learning experiences and environment of one group that makes up a large contingent of the student body in these areas of training as confirmed by college tutors and managers. Drawing on this research and the extensive quotes relating to the experiences and perceptions of tutors and students, the next section teases out the regulatory elements of behaviour, speech, body and sexuality in mothers' body training.

'The means of correct training'

Behaviour

> Obviously they've got to have a certain behaviour, you know, to work towards other people. (Tutor, Waxing)

Training to work on and with other bodies requires certain behaviour – behaviour that is controlled, disciplined and refined. This was manifest in discussion with all tutors and is clearly evidenced in the detailed relaying of an incident by a social care college tutor:

> One of the students in this First Steps [into Care] course, a couple of weeks ago,
> just before we were about to start the lesson, [she was] walking through the corridor,
> and somebody pick-pocketed her purse out of her . . . and she said to me, this had
> happened, so we walked down the corridor, and she saw the girl . . . and then they
> suddenly . . . they erupted into a great big argument and screaming and shouting,
> and if they could have got close to each other, they'd have been ripping their hair
> out and that . . . I suppose, being a registered nurse, it's like so many other
> professions . . . you know, you have to behave in a certain way in and out of work.
> (Tutor, Social Care)

In this example, it is not just what is said, but the physicality of such behaviour with the student behaving in a threatening way. Inappropriate movements and reactions on her part are at odds with the expectations of someone deemed appropriate for nursing. Violence is constructed as the antithesis to caring and the transition to a caring self.

The discourse of 'professionalism' pervades the body training process and early on in courses tutors stress its importance: 'how they [the students] need to conduct themselves and how they need to manage themselves professionally' (Tutor, Waxing) in order to become practitioners. In a Foucauldian power-knowledge circuit (Gordon 1988), this discourse is reverently referred to in order to construct new professional bodies deemed necessary in late modernity for relaying health and social care in the workplace (Dean 2000). But in spite of this, the move towards professionalism can go unheeded and be resisted, sometimes in incidents unrelated to the learning process as above, but very often directly relating to course duties and expectations:

> There was one student in our class that had a bad morning and she'd had some clients booked in, I won't mention any names, and she had a bad attitude from the beginning. Teacher said your client's downstairs and she said I don't need that, I'm not doing that. (Samantha, Beauty Therapy)

By refusing to work on a client and being impolite to the tutor, the student evades the basics of client-focused learning by resisting their presence. The student resists the transition to the working environment and concomitant professional identity.

In an appraisal of Hochshild's writing, Brook (2009) questions whether workers are rendered powerless when undertaking emotional labour and argues that there is more scope for readings of resistance and subversion. We can find such alternate readings at various points in the training experience. For example, in addition to such direct confrontation, there are more subtle and less direct evasions of professional behaviour through imbuing the classroom with a sense of fun and bringing in identities other than that of learner and student. As previously mentioned in relation to the varied uses of training, many of the women we spoke to explained that the classroom was also a social space, and talked of meeting and chatting with friends:

> Sometimes we forget about class and we have fun and we talk and compare things you know which is good. (Fatima, First Steps into Care)

For example, in classes dominated by mothers, discussion provided both a link to and an escape from family responsibilities. In this way, the training space is a contested terrain as tutors and students negotiate the imposed strictures of training behaviour.

Speech
Training to work in close proximity to others' bodies requires careful communication and, in the first instance, this is through speech. The role of verbal communication and the development of client-, patient- or child-focused attentiveness skills are of principal importance and are learned in tandem with the more substantive focus of the courses. Several tutors noted the need for students to overcome shyness and gain confidence in verbal communication, reflecting the need to teach them *how* to speak:

> They are so shy and you can almost see that they are not going to do it because they are so, so shy and reserved, inward . . . it's our job to try and you know get their personality out of them by making them feel safe and happy. (Tutor, Indian Head Massage and Beauty Therapy)

This can be linked to the fact that many of the mothers taking these body training courses were (re)entering education after a considerable period of childcare. But this was also related closely to language capabilities and the fact that, given that the catchment areas of the colleges and the training courses are dominated by new migrants and those with previous low levels of qualification, there were a large number of women with inadequate literacy skills. Some tutors were strict at ensuring that students spoke English, with one perceived problem being the propensity of students to break into language groupings, hindering communication:

I'm trying to get them to speak English, speak English all the time . . . I've actually paired them off with somebody who doesn't speak their language . . . and told them to spend time together in a rather autocratic way . . . but it seems to have worked. (Tutor, Care Studies)

Allied to this and further flagging 'problems' of ethnicity was the suggestion that some students should change the way they spoke, which can be interpreted as a requirement to become more British and fit in with British norms. In the example below, the student is told she needs to tone down both her body language and verbal delivery before working within a childcare context:

Congo people go, da, da, da, da, da [talking very quickly and loudly] . . . My teacher, she said Clarissa, you are rude! (Clarissa, Pathway to Care with ESOL)

On other courses, the speed of speech needed to be regulated:

Talking should be slow and not disturb others. (Tutor, Massage and Reflexology)

This was to ensure the intimacy of working one-on-one and in close proximity to another. This needed to be coupled with a cheerful disposition, as mentioned in the curing focus group, for example, by greeting with a smile, and being polite and friendly. The role of speech is deemed necessary for a confident relationship:

Making them feel confident in you. You know, greeting them with a smile . . . giving them a very friendly manner and polite.

It's making them feel special. (Focus Group, Curing)

In addition to learning the strictures of how to talk, students also need to learn what to say. Most tutors spoke of the need to control the content of talk and, in the first instance, not expressing personal opinions:

I do sometimes look at these people and think . . . oh, goodness me, they're never going to be a nurse or a social worker, because of the views they express. (Tutor, Social Care)

Only vetted professional opinions are acceptable, with some students leaving tutors exasperated by their views. But whereas hairdressing students were encouraged to talk, in other subject areas, such as massage, they were taught to refrain from conversation and use closed questions to keep talk to a minimum. Students needed to learn and negotiate the personal-impersonal in conversation, with students expected to maintain 'professional' and thus impersonal distance.

Body – dress/appearance

The 'right' body is also necessary for embodied practice – whether in the classroom, salon or on placement. The tutor is responsible for enforcing bodily appearance as a literal display of this professionalism. Uniforms are the clearest marker of this and are perceived as important in mirroring the 'cleanness' – in a conceptual as well as a material sense – of the practice to be learned. Except for the care courses, the other courses examined here required students to turn up to class wearing a uniform, normally either of black or white:

> For this sort of field, you've got to look the part, you know, so you've got to look sort of smart and clean, you know, clean and everything tidy, or someone will come in and think, oh! [denoting disdain] . . . (Tutor, Massage and Reflexology)

In our class observations, however, we found this to be personalised through variations in style and with the wearing of jewellery and extra layers, marking out individuality:

> Yeah there's a couple of girls that don't stick to the codes, they come in with things in their hair or whatever and [Tutor, Aromatherapy] will tell them off. (Vicky, Aromatherapy)

Whilst tolerated in theory-based sessions, these additions are frowned upon by tutors in practical sessions as students are visible beyond the student group. In these settings compliance with professional embodiment is required and students are assessed on 'image' before being allowed to proceed with treatment.

It is not only uniform that matters, but ensuring other embodied aspects are tamed and kept in order. Partly, this is to ensure an appealing aesthetic for clients:

> Obviously you have to look clean and the hair's styled nicely, so the clients can look at you and see oh you are really a hairdresser. (Monique and Rupal, Hairdressing)

But as many students on all the courses noted, through a discourse of health and safety, earrings were to be taken out, nails kept short and hair tied back. In relation to the latter this meant that 'inappropriate' touch – in this example between hair and the client body – is prevented:

> You have to have your hair off your face, obviously because if you were doing a massage, or if you are leaning over someone's face they don't want your hair . . . it's not very hygienic you know. No your hair must be back. All earrings must be out. (Vera, Aromatherapy)

Those on care courses, where there did not exist a uniform, again interpreted dress codes through a discourse of professionalism and health and safety, with no high heels, comfortable clothing and minimal jewellery. In relation to direct touching and cleaning aspects of their work, further requirements of dress were required:

> Well you have a dress code regarding when you are changing a child is to apply rubber clothes, plastic apron . . . it's a clean apron every time, disposable ones and gloves, disposable gloves every time. So yeah. (Saadiyah, Childcare)

As Twigg (2000a: 391) points out in relation to dematerialising tendencies within body work, 'status in a profession is marked by distance from the bodily'. With the corporeal processes of touch central to the courses examined here, uniforms and 'protective' clothing are hugely important in their professionalising role and for moving beyond a focus purely on the bodily. Moreover, as indicated below, dress and appearance are directly linked to the desexualisation of the body being trained.

Body – movement/contact

According to Foucault (1977), a disciplined body is the prerequisite of an efficient gesture. Training for body work requires the learning and, in some instances, the constant repetition of movements and actions. As Lea (2009: 473) articulates in relation to Thai yoga massage, embodied knowledge is not simply about remembering and then doing, but 'considering the (inter-personal and inter-corporeal) relation set up between the massage practitioner and recipient'. Bodily co-ordination is vital. One tutor here, who teaches hairdressing, felt that this could not always be taught and hence wanted one student with improper movements removed from her class:

> In hairdressing, if you cannot co-ordinate, it means that you cannot carry out a physical task, because you cannot co-ordinate yourself to be able to carry that out in a healthy and a safe way, so you're endangering your clients' welfare . . . this course is not suitable for her, because she can't follow instructions, she cannot co-ordinate. (Tutor, Hairdressing)

Learning embodied knowledge crucially requires a spatial ordering of one body in relation to another. As one student on the massage course remarked: 'They explain to us about all of that, the professional Code of Conduct and you have to be careful how you lean over the client, you've got to behave in a professional manner' (Vicky, Massage). The setting of bodily boundaries through touch and proximity and, conversely, avoidance and distance is, again, couched through a discourse of professionalism and requires a self-reflexive process by the student (Gale 2009). Negotiating this 'dialectic of distance and intimacy' (Churchill and Churchill 1982) is essential. For one pregnant mother, this issue came to the fore through changes to her own body:

> A couple of weeks before we stopped and then [Tutor, Aromatherapy] says 'you're not massaging' and I thought 'oi, I can stand up, just'. And she goes 'no your belly is getting in the way'. I goes 'it's not getting in the way yet'. (Annie, Aromatherapy)

The gradual yet increasingly pronounced touch of her stomach with the bodies of her clients disrupts initial and prescribed bodily boundaries. The growing pregnant body, through inappropriate touch, becomes matter out of place in the training environment (Longhurst 2000) and as the training process develops. Moreover, as her pregnant body grew, the student could no longer fit into her uniform, further marking her as 'other' and further distancing her from the regulated embodied practice of the classroom.

Students on the majority of these courses also have to 'practise' their learning and often on a range of different bodies. But whilst these courses trade on this embodied encounter of touch, they also require the controlling and disguising of feelings towards others' bodies. For some students, there was resistance to working on or with certain bodies – most especially seen on several courses in relation to particular ethnicities and religious beliefs and working with men's bodies. This was interpreted as an issue of attitude according to the care studies tutor:

> It's a question of attitude . . . so I have to say, well, you know, if you really do feel like that, I'm afraid it's no point in thinking of going into nursing, no point at all, because you will have to work with men and women. (Tutor, Care Studies)

This again raises questions of how gender intersects with ethnicity and religious beliefs and their interpretation, and the extent to which embodied regulation and requirements are prepared to be met.

In relation to reflexology, students spoke about encountering smelly feet or older people's feet (which were considered the most disgusting) and how they need to keep in check their responses, offering a 'professional' line:

> I think by the time you take up reflexology you have to like, you have to be prepared to touch anybody's feet so. Most people are like 'ah' [sounds disgusted] at the beginning so... (Focus Group, Curing)

> Yeah I mean if it was really bad you couldn't stand it you can suggest politely that you go and have a little wash but obviously in a very tactful sort of way. . . . Yeah, yeah that's mentioned yeah. You wouldn't say 'hey your feet stink'. (Focus Group, Curing)

However, interviews demonstrated that this was not sustained in the client's and tutor's absence with, for example, massage students joking about particular clients whose bodies behaved in ways deemed inappropriate or were seen as problematic.

Scott (1990) stresses the importance of analysing the 'hidden transcripts' of resistance, the 'hidden' acts of protest that take place 'offstage' and beyond the direct observation of those in authority. From these examples, we see how students are expected to give a professional response to what are embodied encounters with so-called 'problem' bodies, though still resisting this fully professional identity by laughing about clients in their absence. This again can be construed as a distancing from the bodily (Twigg 2000a) – or, more accurately, a distancing from perceived problematic bodies. So whilst the expressions of the student are governed by the rules of learning, in the absence of the client and tutor, these are resisted.

Sexuality
Marcuse (1968 cited in Gimlin 2007) argued that embodied displays of sexuality are encouraged by employers as a means of gratification in otherwise mundane jobs. In contrast, in body training any hint of sexuality is hidden away with the active avoidance of any possible trace of its presence in these types of work.

In relation to care, and especially childcare, bodily boundaries were commonly discussed early on in the training course with tutors and students at pains to point out appropriate and inappropriate embodied interactions to deter claims of child abuse:

> Especially when we have more policies and regulations to follow you know for example you can't put children on your lap and give them a cuddle and a kiss you know. (Tutor, Pre-school practice)

However, as the tutor here explains, this is perceived as requiring a tempering of seemingly natural maternal behaviour in the care of children.

With other types of training, notably in massage, there is a purposeful desexualisation of the environment and students to offset the widespread connections made between it and sex work:

> You don't want you know, to be misconstrued, you know, it's your job. (Tutor, Aromatherapy)

Among the mothers discussed here and as mentioned earlier, being in training was seen as a 'respectable' position and correct and properly worn uniform came to the fore in terms of promoting respectability in relation to desexualisation. This was highlighted by the waxing tutor:

> Little things like, I spoke to them about, making sure that their uniform was correct, so making sure things like, that their clothing wasn't too low or revealing, that the language they're using is very professional and in no way whatsoever suggestive to the client, obviously with male clients especially. (Tutor, Waxing)

So, ensuring the body can be easily read as professional, with no suggestion of anything other, is key. This was reiterated by students, as one remarks in relation to make-up, over-doing it would be considered suggestive, leading to the sexually promiscuous:

> You can wear a little bit of make-up but obviously don't over do it. (Nina, Reflexology)

Bodily presentations have to be kept closely in check, stamping out overt feminine and heterosexual performances.

As Oerton (2004) suggests, women therapeutic workers have to work hard to mark out their professional distance from clients by deploying professional identification by using boundary-setting devices or techniques. As society has become more sexualised, steps are taken in therapeutic work to remove itself from this sexualisation, with 'professional' appearance through uniform and look constantly re-enforced. The aforementioned setting of bodily boundaries is, again, couched through a discourse of professionalism and requires a self-regulatory and reflexive process by the student. For massage, this was relayed in relation to the sensitivities of dealing with male clients as this tutor suggests:

> And we teach them with a man, how to approach the man because certain areas in a man can be stimulated more easily than a woman so we teach them all those things. (Tutor, Massage and Reflexology)

As bodily displays of sexuality are considered an incursion into these therapeutic spaces, students need to learn quickly the right balance between closeness and distance and learn how to respond to the sexual:

> You would say, 'right, turn over and we'll work on your back'. (Vera, aromatherapy massage).

With nakedness at odds with social mores and expectations where the body is hidden and out of sight, here, it is the role of the student to control what is seen and touched. This reiterates Twigg's (2006) discussion of what is acceptable and unacceptable in body work, with an embodied gradient of touch relating to the human body and its location.

Conclusions: the body-body articulation

In discussing the role of the control of activity in the production of docile bodies, one element Foucault stresses is the body-object articulation. Here, discipline identifies the relationship between the body and the object that it manipulates, embracing as it does the whole body:

> Over the whole surface of contact between the body and the object it handles, power is introduced, fastening them to one another . . . The regulation imposed by power is at the same time the law of construction of operation. (1977: 153)

This is a relationship that requires the body and its gestures to be broken down in minute and determined ways.

By exploring the process of training for body work among mothers, this relationship of power and its concomitant disciplinary procedures is relevant, though it falls some way short in understanding the necessary body-body articulation that is being examined here. In this chapter we have traced some of the regulatory elements of body training and the processes through which students are turned into body workers. With a focus on behaviour, speech, body and sexuality, this close body-body contact of interacting body work requires initial bodily manipulation and constant monitoring in order to provide professional skill and care.

Many of the regulatory examples we draw on here are not particular to women or mothers. There exists, however, a gendered trace of regulation with a tempering of certain constructed feminine performances and identities. This is seen most especially in efforts to render invisible the sexually marked female body and presumed heterosexual identity – whether this be embodied through pregnancy or marked through dress and make-up. Conversely, there is also a need to repeal the perceived innate or developed maternal caring self through constant recourse to the professionalisation of these varied body training subject areas. The female body needs to be constantly kept in check.

Focusing on the liminal 'in between' space of training, these processes of creating a professional identity and body are not straightforward. Instead, as students emerge from the classroom, to practise in the salon or during placement, there are a number of points for resistance or subversion in the learning process as students exercise their agency. Thus, the transition from student to potential worker carrying a particular professional identity is not always a smooth and straightforward process.

What this chapter also flags up is the resonance and usefulness of the concept of body work to focus on the interaction between bodies. As mentioned at the outset, the courses studied here are broad in scope, covering varied health, beauty and social care subjects. These courses and the work they lead to are quite different in terms of purpose, content and setting. In spite of this, however, a close examination of the training process highlights a number of convergences round the expectations of behaviour, speech, body and sexuality, which bind them together, at least in relation to the cohort of students explored here. This suggests the usefulness of exploring diverse examples of training and work for their bodily and embodied dimensions under the rubric of body work, although these comparative dimensions warrant further interest.

As a final comment, and to link back to the pervasive policy context of training for work in the UK, body training can be seen as a paradoxical space (Rose 1993) and learning process – one of regulation and entrenched stereotypes, but also of new possibilities and self-determination. As has been the focus of this chapter, training is aimed at transforming students' bodies and minds through instruction and discipline to service and care for particular client and patient groups in very specific ways. Yet, at the same time, it trades on the stereotyping of women's and mothers' skills and training abilities which is decidedly problematic. For example, the Women and Work Commission has recently reported that girls and women are still being encouraged to pursue 'traditional' jobs (Women and Work Commission 2009) where pay remains low. Education is considered 'critical' by the Commission in breaking down these gender stereotypes and closing the pay gap, yet training for body work still falls back on notions of what are deemed compatible jobs for women and mothers. This needs to be more thoroughly challenged. However, training can provide these students with confidence, language and communication skills, and embodied expertise. These learning experiences can thus open up new personal, employment and financial possibilities. To return to Foucault, this paradoxical space and learning process can be interpreted through his productive notion of disciplinary power. As he suggests: 'power . . . exerts a positive influence on life, that endeavours to administer, optimise, and multiply it, subjecting it to precise controls and comprehensive regulations' (Foucault 1979: 3).

Acknowledgements

This chapter is based on research funded by the ESRC (RES-061-23-0106). We are indebted to all those who participated in the study, most especially the mothers who gave up their time to participate in focus groups and interviews. Thanks to reviewers for valuable comments and particular thanks to the editorial team for their suggestions and encouragement.

Notes

1   This notion of 'non-working' stems from Governmental definitions and refers to being outside paid employment. We recognise that this is highly problematic, given it ignores non-paid work that mothers undertake in the home.
2   The chapter by Wainwright et al. (2010, Geoforum) draws on the performativity of gender and maternal identity in the choosing of body training courses and hence these Butler-inspired arguments are not repeated in this chapter.
3   Further details of the project can be found at: http://www.brunel.ac.uk/about/acad/sse/chg/projects/body
4   We use these terms merely as a means of initial categorisation and an aid to the research process. We therefore acknowledge that the subject areas they include are overlapping and entangled.

References

Acker, J. (1990) Hierarchies, jobs, bodies: a theory of gendered organisations, Gender and Society, 4, 139–58.
Appleby, Y. and Bathmaker, A. (2006) The new skills agenda: increased lifelong learning or new sites of inequality? British Educational Research Journal, 32, 703–17.
Brook, P. (2009) The alienated heart: Hochschild's emotional labour thesis and the anti-capitalist politics of alienation, Capital and Class, 98, 7–31.
Brush, L. (1999) Gender, work, who cares?! Production, reproduction, deindustrialisation, and business as usual. In Feree, M.M., Lober, J. and Hess, B. (eds) Revisioning Gender. London: Sage.
Buckingham, S., Marandet, E., Smith, F., Wainwright, E. and Diosi, M. (2006) The liminality of training spaces: places of public / private transitions, Geoforum, 37, 895–905.
Churchill, L.R. and Churchill, S.W. (1982) Storytelling in medical arenas: the art of self-determination, Literature and Medicine, 1, 73–9.
Davidson, J. and Milligan, C. (2004) Editorial: Embodying emotion sensing space: introducing emotional geographies, Social and Cultural Geography, 5, 523–32.

Dean, H. (2000) Introduction: Towards an embodied account of welfare. In Ellis, K. and Dean, H. (eds) *Social Policy and the Body: Transitions in Corporeal Discourse*. Basingstoke: Macmillan.

Department for Education and Employment (2001) *Skills for Life, The National Strategy for Improving Adult Literacy and Numeracy Skills*. London: Stationery Office.

Dyer, S., McDowell, L. and Batnitzky, A. (2008) Emotional labour / body work: the caring labours of migrants in the UK's National Health Service, *Geoforum*, 39, 2030–38.

Evans, R. and Thomas, F. (2009) Emotional interactions and ethics of care: caring for a family member with HIV and AIDS, *Emotion, Space and Society*, 2, 111–9.

Foucault, M. (1977) *Discipline and Punish: the Birth of the Prison*. London: Penguin.

Foucault, M. (1979) *The History of Sexuality, Volume 1: The Will to Knowledge*. London: Penguin.

Gale, N. (2007) *Knowing the Body and Embodying Knowledge: an Ethnography of Student Practitioner Experiences in Osteopathy and Homeopathy*. Unpublished PhD thesis, University of Warwick.

Gale, N. (2009) Promoting patient-practitioner partnership in clinical training, *Learning in Health and Social Care*, 8, 13–21.

Gimlin, D. (1996) Pamela's place: power and negotiation in the hair salon, *Gender and Society*, 10, 505–26.

Gimlin, D. (2007) What is body work? A review of literature, *Sociology Compass*, 353–70.

Gordon, C. (ed.) (1988) *Power/knowledge: Selected Interviews and other Writings 1972–1977*. New York: Pantheon.

Halford, S., Witz, A. and Savage, M. (1997) *Gender, Careers and Organisations*. Basingstoke: MacMillan.

Hochschild, A. (1983) *The Managed Heart: Commercialisation of Human Feeling*. Los Angeles: University of California Press.

Kang, M. (2003) The managed hand: the commercialisation of bodies and emotions in Korean immigrant-owned nail salons, *Gender and Society*, 17, 820–39.

Lea, J. (2009) Bridging skills: the geographies of teaching and learning embodied knowledges, *Geoforum*, 40, 465–74.

Longhurst, R. (2000) Corporeographies of pregnancy: 'bikini babes', *Environment and Planning D*, 18, 453–72.

McDowell, L. (1997) *Capital Culture: Gender at Work in the City*. Oxford: Blackwell-Wiley.

McDowell, L. (2009) *Working Bodies: Interactive Service Employment and Workplace Identities*. Oxford: Blackwell-Wiley.

McDowell, L. and Court, G. (1994) Performing work: bodily representations in merchant banks, *Environment and Planning D*, 12, 253–78.

McDowell, L., Ray, K., Perrons, D., Fagan, C. and Ward, K. (2005a) Women's paid work and moral economies of care, *Social and Cultural Geography*, 6, 219–35.

McDowell, L., Perrons, D., Fagan, C., Ray, K. and Ward, K. (2005b) The contradictions and intersections of class and gender in a global city: placing working women's lives on the research agenda, *Environment and Planning A*, 37, 441–61.

Milligan, C. (2000) Bearing the burden: towards a restructured geography of caring, *Area*, 32, 49–58.

Milligan, C. (2003) Location or dis-location: from community to long-term care – the caring experience, *Social and Cultural Geography*, 4, 455–70.

O'Connor, H. and Madge, C. (2005) Mothers in the making? Exploring liminality in cyber / space, *Transactions of the Institute of British Geographers, NS* 30, 83–97.

Oerton, S. (2004) Bodywork boundaries: power, politics and professionalism in therapeutic spaces, *Gender, Work and Organization*, 11, 544–65.

Osgood, J. (2005) Who cares? The classed nature of childcare, *Gender and Education*, 17, 289–303.

Paterson, M. (2007) *The Senses of Touch: Haptics, Affects and Technologies*. Oxford: Berg.

Pratt, G. (2002) Studying immigrants in focus groups. In Moss, P. (ed.) *Feminist Geography in Practice: Research and Methods*. Oxford: Blackwell.

Pratt, G. (2004) *Working Feminism*. Edinburgh: Edinburgh University Press.

Rose, G. (1993) *Feminism and Geography: the Limits of Geographical Knowledge*. Cambridge: Polity.

Scott, J. (1990) *Domination and the Arts of Resistance: Hidden Transcripts*. Newhaven: Yale University Press.

Sharma, U. and Black, P. (2001) Look good, feel better: beauty therapy as emotional labour, *Sociology*, 35, 4, 913–31.

Shields, R. (1991) *Places on the Margin: Alternative Geographies of Modernity*. London: Routledge.

Shilling, C. (1993) *The Body and Social Theory*. London: Sage.

Simpson, R. (2004) Masculinity at work: the experiences of men in female dominated occupations, *Work, Employment and Society*, 18, 349–68.

Skeggs, B. (1997) *Formations of Class and Gender*. London: Sage.

Smith, D. (1988) *The Everyday World as Problematic*. Boston: Northeastern University Press.

Smith, F., Barker, J., Wainwright, E., Marandet, E. and Buckingham, S. (2008) A new deal for lone parents? Training lone parents for work in West London, *Area*, 40, 237–44.

Tretheway, A. (1999) Disciplined bodies: women's embodied identities at work, *Organisation Studies*, 20, 423–50.

Turner, V. (1982) *From Ritual to Theatre: the Human Seriousness of Play*. New York: PAJ Publications.

Twigg, Julia (2000a) Carework as a form of bodywork, *Ageing and Society*, 20, 389–411.

Twigg, Julia (2000b) *Bathing: the Body and Community Care*. London: Routledge.

Twigg, J. (2006) *The Body in Health and Social Care*. Hampshire: Palgrave Macmillan.

van Dongen, E. and Elema, R. (2001) The art of touching: the culture of 'body work' in nursing, *Anthropology and Medicine*, 8, 149–62.

Wainwright, E., Buckingham, S., Marandet, E. and Smith, F. (2010) Body training: investigating the embodied training choices of/for mothers in West London, *Geoforum*, 41, 489–97.

Wainwright, E., Marandet, E., Buckingham, S. and Smith, F. (in press a) Mothers' participation in and progression through the neo-liberal learning market, *Gender, Place and Culture*.

Wainwright, E., Marandet, E., Rizvi, S. and Smith, F. (in press b) The microgeographies of learning bodies and emotions in the 'classroom-salon', *Emotion, Space and Society*.

Williams, S. (1998) Capitalising on emotions? Re-thinking the inequalities in the health debate, *Sociology*, 32, 12–39.

Wolkowitz, C. (2002) The social relations of body work, *Work, Employment and Society*, 16, 497–510.

Wolkowitz, C. (2006) *Bodies at Work*. London: Sage.

Women and Work Commission (2009) *Shaping a Fairer Future: a Review of the Recommendations of the Women and Work Commission Three Years On*. London: Stationery Office.

Young, I. (1990) *Throwing Like a Girl and Other Essays in Feminist Philosophy and Social Theory*. Indiana University Press, Indiana.

5

From body-talk to body-stories: body work in complementary and alternative medicine
Nicola Kay Gale

Introduction

This chapter explores the 'body work' undertaken by practitioners of complementary and alternative medicine (CAM), in the light of ethnographic research on the education of practitioners in two contrasting disciplines: osteopathy and homeopathy. Body work refers to a (growing) employment sector where the work involves distinctive and often intimate relations with the bodies of the consumers, clients or patients (Wolkowitz 2006: 18–19). Gimlin (2007) has noted that one of the most common uses of the term 'body work' in the sociological literature has been to refer to 'labour performed on behalf of or directly on other people's bodies' (2007: 358). The sociology of health and illness has provided an understandable home for many sociologists interested in the body and embodiment. Sociological research has brought many insights into the ways in which, in medical work, the body is conceptualised as an 'object' of medical knowledge, and embedded in a dualist (Cartesian) framework that separates mind from body and places them in an asymmetric power relationship. However, the focus on the sick bodies on which healthcare work is performed paints only a partial picture, because it does not fully recognise the interactional nature of consultations, which also requires that practitioners are able to negotiate their own (precarious) embodiment in the therapeutic relationship (Cassell 1998, Lawler 1991).

CAM practitioners are an interesting case through which to investigate the concept of body work, first, because the philosophies that underlie CAM practices are often different from biomedicine, in terms of articulating 'holistic' or 'naturalistic' models of the body in health and illness[1]. For instance, CAM practitioners often hyphenate 'dis-ease' to emphasise the emotional and social components of illness. Secondly, CAM clients have distinctive experiences of treatment, for instance developing a 'fresh and sustained sense of bodily responsibility that induces new health practices' (Baarts and Pedersen 2009: 1) and having a more 'active' role in the management of illness in the pursuit of health (Sharma 1992). This begs the question of what *work* practitioners are doing to play their part in bringing about these new practices and perceptions and how the 'body' and embodiment of those on both sides of the therapeutic encounter are managed. The educational environment provides an ideal location for exploring the philosophical and practical assumptions that underpin day- to-day practice. As students experience the struggle and awkwardness of learning new skills and knowledge, it brings issues of the embodied intersubjectivity between practitioners and patients into sharp relief.

This chapter begins by summarising the methodological approach that I used to research the embodied experiences of the student-practitioners. Unconventionally perhaps, I do not start with an in-depth literature review but I present the data first 'on their own terms' (although you will note occasional references to literature where there are interesting parallels to be seen). These data relate to osteopaths' and homeopaths' experiences of learning to communicate with, touch and facilitate the healing process for their embodied patients (a stage roughly equivalent to case-taking and diagnosis in conventional medical treatment). Students develop an understanding of the healing process as it is conceptualised in the osteopathic and homeopathic models and, as well as learning to interact with the bodies of their patients, they develop a new orientation to their own bodies. Indeed, their own embodiment is made explicit in the learning environment. By drawing and critically exploring key sociological concepts of the body and embodiment, reflexivity and narrative in the light of the data, I argue that the dialogical construction of body-stories challenges Cartesian dualism. Finally, I discuss what the data might mean for the future development of the sociological concept of 'body work'.

Studying CAM student practitioners

The data presented in the chapter were collected through ethnographic research conducted in two case study educational institutions in England, the anonymised College of Osteopathy and College of Homeopathy. The College of Osteopathy runs a four-year full-time course and the College of Homeopathy a three-year part-time course. Although both colleges train practitioners who are amongst the more 'professionalised' CAM groups[2], the case studies provide a good contrast with each other: osteopathy involves structural adjustments directly on the physical body while the homeopathic consultation is primarily talk-based, with the administration of a 'remedy' that the patient usually takes at home. As I will argue below, despite the absence of physical touch in the latter practice, the bodies of both the practitioner and the patient are central to the interactions and work that take place in both. It is important to note, however, that the details of the curriculum are not necessarily representative of education in the wider profession: there is much variation in training, especially in homeopathy which is not statutorily regulated.

The choice of ethnographic methods was motivated by epistemological and ethical considerations. Although I was familiar with the field of CAM through previous research and as a user, I was concerned that because CAM is socially excluded from mainstream biomedical healthcare practice, it was important to understand the culture from within (Gale 2010). Ethnography, with its rich history of the anthropological study of 'other' cultures (Geertz 1973, Malinowski 1922) and sociological study of sub-cultures (Bulmer 1984), seemed an appropriate method. I sought to immerse myself in the two professional cultures and, as Barrett (2000) calls for, to try to retain some of the passion of the field by having 'more respect for other ideas on their own terms, not translated into [sociology's] own' and to 'appeal to experience beyond cognition' (Barrett 2000: 20). However, it was fruitful throughout to think about the difference between the 'body' (as one part of Cartesian mind/body dualism) and 'embodiment' (phenomenological lived body/self) and ways in which the work of these CAM practitioners challenges existing sociological theory and concepts, particularly the idea of the 'body'.

Over one academic year, I spent approximately 200 hours in each college, taking part in classes, clinics and social activities. My focus was on exploring how these students learn to undertake the work they do and how different ways of knowing are valued in the training. The findings presented in this chapter are primarily based on data from classroom encounters, rather than the student clinics where students come into contact with real patients. Classroom teaching, inevitably, avoids many of the uncertainties of clinical training, and so can tend to reproduce 'ideal' models of the healing process and the therapeutic encounter. Some of the challenges that students face in maintaining theory in practice in the student clinics, with the dual constraints of care of the patient and demonstrating their learning and skills to pass the course, have been reported elsewhere (Gale 2008). It was not possible to get formal ethical approval for the study, as there was no system at the university at the time. I did, however, have my protocol peer-reviewed and negotiated carefully with both of the Colleges, explaining what I was doing and how the data collected would be used. I then obtained a mixture of written and oral consent from students to participate in their classes, assuring anonymity, that participation was voluntary and that they could withdraw at any time. Mindful of issues of harm, and understanding that an excluded group of healthcare professionals may have legitimate concerns about the impact of the research, I often engaged in discussions about the research and its implications with my participants throughout the study (for more detail, see Gale 2010).

Osteopathy and homeopathy

Before I begin presenting the data, it may be useful to quickly sketch the theory underpinning the two practices. Osteopathy was developed by an American physician, Andrew Taylor Still (1828–1917), whose research involved the detailed study of human anatomy, and he ultimately concluded that if the structure (especially the bones) of the body was not aligned correctly, it would impede its functions. As the body was understood as naturally self-healing, any dysfunction could have far-reaching effects on many systems of the body, leading to disease. Tenderness, restriction, asymmetry and tissue texture change are signs of poor *adaptation* of the body to external events. Diagnosis is not a single event, but 'the long term development of an integrative and dynamic model' of the person's mal/functioning (McKone 2001: 236) and treatment attempts to restore function.

Homeopathy was founded by a German physician and chemist, Samuel Hahnemann (1755–1843), who, while undertaking exploratory research into the action of pharmaceutical herbs and chemicals, observed that if given in a minute dose, a substance (usually plant, mineral or animal) can cure the same symptoms that in a material dose it would produce – known as the principle of 'like cures like' (*similia similibus curantur*). For example, the homeopathic 'remedy' *Belladonna* (deadly nightshade), which in material doses would cause fever and ultimately death, can be given for fever symptoms. Each remedy has a constellation of physical, mental, emotional, social and environmental symptoms/characteristics associated with it, and the goal of the homeopathic consultation is to find the remedy that is the most similar to the patient's experiences. The process of 'potentisation' used to 'dilute' substances used in homeopathy is highly controversial in conventional medical science as it sits in direct opposition to the current dominant scientific paradigm (Kuhn 1962) of the way that the body works, based on chemistry and pharmacology. In homeopathic theory, so- called 'symptoms' are not signs of the disease (as in biomedical theory) but they are aspects of the body's own healing process at work, in its attempts to restore balance to the human system. Interventions should catalyse or energise this process when it has become stuck or slow through a weakening of the 'vital force' (which is a concept similar to the Chinese *chi*).

From body-talk to body-stories

During the course, students in both the Colleges of Osteopathy and Homeopathy learn firstly, ways of listening to the embodied patient and, secondly, ways of analysing how to treat the dis-eased body. I explore these two aspects of their work using the emergent concepts of *body-talk* and *body-stories*, neither of which are *in vivo* concepts but which are useful to bring together and theorise actors' explanations and my observations on learning about the healing process and the work of these practitioners.

Learning to listen to body-talk

For the student practitioners, learning to listen to body-talk is an important clinical task, and one that is fundamentally embodied and intersubjective. Body-talk describes the ways in which the embodied patient is able to communicate with the practitioner. This dialogical character of the therapeutic encounter captures explicitly the idea of an active patient.

Osteopathy
The student-osteopaths learn three main ways to listen to body-talk: oral case-taking, observation and touch (palpation). The development of palpatory skills (to palpate is to touch as part of a physical examination) is assigned the most time and value within the course because touch is seen as the cornerstone of osteopathic practice.

Oral case-taking is taught through role-play (before students take cases in clinic) and the students' skills of verbal interaction gradually become more effective and efficient for obtaining the information that they require. This is perhaps the most obvious way in which an embodied patient is able to communicate his or her ill health – through a linguistic representation of dis-ease, usually either in narrative form or as a direct response to questioning. The student-osteopaths learn to use a very tightly structured patient information sheet to record information about the patient, which while it inevitably affects the way they elicit patients' experiences also ensures that they get a lot of detail about all aspects of the person's health (not just their presenting complaint).

Learning *palpation* requires both an academic knowledge of anatomy/physiology and physical motor skills. At an embodied level, each student must integrate what Belenky *et al.* (1997) term banker-teaching (the conventional mode of imparting knowledge to students) and midwife-teaching (apprenticeship and drawing knowledge out from students). This process is carefully staged at the College, with the academic knowledge forefronted. During the four years, students 'get a feel' for the structures of the body through classes that involve touching bone specimens and where they practise techniques on each others' bodies. They first familiarise themselves with 'normally' functioning bones and tissues (muscles, fascia and to a lesser extent viscera), then explore what dysfunction (dis-ease) feels like. As they progress through the course, they are encouraged to adapt the techniques they have learnt to the specific requirements of each patient and their own body's characteristics and capabilities. One tutor explained that it is much better to enter into 'a dialogue with the tissues, so that you are constantly assessing, then treating, then assessing, then treating and so on'. This language used – 'dialogue' – highlights the extent to which osteopathic treatment happens at the point of interaction between two embodied agents, rather than being simply imposed on a passive patient's body.

Some observations such as the 'quality' of movement or of tissues – aspects of what the body can communicate to the osteopath – are not easily translatable in these anatomical terms. Tutors sometime use metaphor 'a beach ball in the water and you are trying to push it underwater and it is resisting' but often just have to demonstrate what you 'do' and get the students to feel it for themselves as this excerpt from field notes shows:

> The tutor's eyes seemed to glaze over when she was demonstrating the technique. She had to stop what she was doing to explain to the observing students what they would have to do to get the technique right. While she was actually feeling for the tissues and locating her own hands and body in relation to the body of the student model, she seemed entirely focused at the point of bodily interaction. But for her students, it was necessary for her to take a step back and orientate them.

The students experience being on both 'sides' of the interaction; as a student explained, 'you have to do it and have it done to you before you try it on a patient'.

The final component of listening to body-talk, *observation*, includes a consideration of factors such as the patient's appearance ('Are they fat and lifeless or fat and vigorous?' 'Self esteem: How might this show?') and whether 'these observations contrast with their spoken story'. Observational skills were generally associated with developing expertise and subtlety of approach; as one tutor asserted, 'The art of observation is key in osteopathy . . . to observe is to become aware through careful attention, for at least a few minutes'. He warned against 'restless hand syndrome – trying to get your big paws on the patient' too quickly.

The triangulation of the three methods demonstrates the centrality of embodied interaction at the investigative stage of the osteopathic healing process. What emerges of interest is, first, that the skills the student osteopaths learn cannot be reduced to language, they are fundamentally embodied; as one student put it, 'you know so many techniques and you don't know how you know them'. Second, practitioner embodiment is an explicit subject of study and attention.

Homeopathy
For the student homeopaths, the body emerges as a 'communicator' with agency not subsumed by or reduced to a mind-directed agency, as these various quotes by College of Homeopathy tutors show:

> The body is intelligent.

> We have forgotten how to listen to our bodies.

> The body is not stupid, it tells you what it needs and says, 'Listen!' If you don't, next time it says it louder.

> From our point of view, the body is *saying* 'Breast Cancer'.

> I always think: What is the body telling me about the self and where I need to do work?

The kind of 'body' that the homeopathy students are working with is not a 'plastic body' that can be readily moulded by advances in biomedical science (*e.g.* Williams and Bendelow 1998: 80). For the homeopaths, medical control over the human body (based on a Cartesian model) is an illusion, because there is a much more fluid and interactional relationship between the body, the emotions, the mind and the social and physical environment. Using this framework, symptoms, behaviours and emotions are a form of body-talk, they are expressions of a state of dis-ease. Rather than disease being a purely negative aspect of life, or a 'disruption' (Bury 1982), homeopaths view illness as a potentially positive force for change, perhaps highlighting aspects of a person's life that were unsustainable or indicating, from a spiritual perspective, that the personality might have taken a path that deviates from the 'soul journey'. As one tutor explained, 'The body is an ally to the soul, not the personality'. It is clear that the concept of the *body* is different from the biomedical body, in that it has agency and is not dualistically subordinated to the mind, but there is also a concern in the homeopathic encounter with *embodiment* and patient experience.

The aim of treatment is to find a remedy that most closely matches the patient's physical, mental, emotional, social and environmental state. In order to do this, the student-homeopaths must learn to build up a detailed, multi-dimensional picture of their patient, including his or her character, likes and dislikes, susceptibilities and aspects of the physical, mental and emotional symptoms, often using the 'CLAMS method' (an acronym for concomitant symptoms, location, aetiology, modalities – what makes the discomfort better or worse – and sensations). Even for emotional symptoms it will be important to ascertain these details, such as where in the body the person feels the emotion. For example, a patient may feel anxiety in their stomach, their throat, or their legs, and this will affect the prescription. This process can also be conceptualised as a combination of three methods: oral case taking, observation and touch (energy work). These methods of listening to body-talk, compared to the osteopaths' methods, are much more interdependent and are taught in an integrated way rather than as separate skills.

Much of the consultation involves eliciting 'talk' from their patient largely in narrative form. A number of tutors regularly asserted that students should think about consultations as '*receiving* a case' rather than 'taking a case', allowing the patient to tell his or her story as much as possible without interruption and recording the patients' own words. However, the listener is not passive, as one tutor said, 'A great skill to acquire as a case-taker is to pursue symptoms. You have to get to the root of them or you end up too general' but he also warned, 'People can be deeply resistant to seeing connections, which can be frustrating, but you have to give people the benefit of the doubt and you have to be self-critical. Try not to read things into a case because it has a connection for you . . . You must respond to where the patient is now or you will miss the similar remedy'. Another tutor told a story to illustrate the importance of effective questioning:

> A patient came to me and she had had weeping ulcers around her right ankle for many years. She had to have regular home visits from a nurse who would redress the ankle. So I thought the right side relates to what has happened to us in a practical sense in our life. And the ankles relate to support. So I asked her, 'How much support do you have in your life?' She broke down into tears for five or six minutes. All I could do at this point was to hug her and wait for her to finish crying. Then when she stopped crying I asked her, 'And how do you feel about that?' and then the anger started to come though. So I gave her a remedy not for ankles or ulcers but for suppressed anger.

The words of the patient, however, should be triangulated with *observations*. The 'way' that the patient conveys his or her story gives additional insights. Thus, a patient who needs the remedy *Thuja* might not finish sentences, change the subject or answer the wrong question (first-year lecture). The value of observation comes not only from recording what actually happens but from what does not or remains unsaid.

Finally, *touch* takes on an unconventional 'energetic' (non-material) form. When the body with dis-ease is understood as more than simply a physical body, touch in the assessment of the patient is similarly not limited to physical touch. Phrases used by tutors to attempt to capture this in words included 'energy', 'holding the space' or 'witnessing'. For example, a tutor explained, 'So often in our practice we have people who come in and tell us things that they have never told anyone before, and you have to hold the space for them to do that'. The language is interesting, as 'holding' implies a physicality to it, yet 'space' is something that cannot really be grasped. There is a physicality to the experience of being with someone, sharing the space of the consultation room and being a witness to their emotions, even without physical contact in the conventional sense. Learning these skills of energetic touch requires a deeply embodied and reflexive approach that nurtures sensitivity to subtle changes in the atmosphere between two people. For instance, in a class on a common remedy called *Staphysagria*, students were invited to give examples of their own experience of taking the remedy. One first-year student spoke movingly about her experiences of miscarriage, while the others listened to her, and after she had finished speaking, the tutor thanked her, and slowly turned to the class and asked, 'Can you feel the energy of *Staphysagria* now?' It is difficult to put words to the atmosphere in the class at the time, because it was a mixture of emotions, such as sadness and grief, experiences, such as violation and pain, and bodily responses, such as tears, but the students responded with 'yes' to the question. Witnessing other students' responses allows each student to stand back from his or her own experience, compare it with that of others, objectify and be reflective about it (*cf*. Crossley 2001: 142). Students are encouraged to explore their personal responses to topics and remedies. One tutor said, 'If you haven't done it yourself, how will you hold the space for someone else?'

Learning to construct body-stories

The concept 'body-story' describes the narrative that is co-constructed by patient and practitioner to explore aetiology and/or the way in which the dis-ease plays a part in their lives. Osteopathy and homeopathy have different approaches to drawing together the aspects of the body-talk into a coherent body-story. Within the scope of this chapter I cannot present a full account of the complex process of narrative construction but, in the context of understanding the nature of the work performed, it is important to compare the construction of the body-story to its approximate equivalent in biomedicine – the 'diagnosis'. While in biomedicine the goal of the consultation is to arrive at a singular disease label (the diagnosis), in these CAM therapies the goal is an understanding of the way that dis-ease has manifested in the body as a response to external and internal disturbances, and how that dis-ease has changed over time to become the embodied distress listened to in the consultation. In addition, while the biomedical diagnosis is a tool in the selection of an appropriate treatment but has no intrinsic role in healing, the construction of the body-story in both homeopathy and osteopathy is also an integral part of the healing process inseparable from the treatment (*i.e.* physical adjustments or homeopathic remedy).

For instance, the student-osteopaths learn specific concepts to elucidate the body-story, such as 'legacy' or 'tissue memory'. Legacy is understood as the totality of people's embodied experiences and is stored in the tissues. Events like emotional or physical trauma can leave traces in the body in terms of tension, pain or habitual behaviour. Tools like time-lines are used by the students to help map out the potentially complex aetiology of the present distress. The following example shows how the process of listening to the body-talk, forming a body-story and treatment are difficult to separate in practice:

> A woman came to me who had been having bad headaches ever since she was mugged. We tried all sorts of treatments, but then I noticed that here [indicates over the student model above her left shoulder] there was a palpable feeling that she was expecting to be hit again. It was about how she was holding herself. So I held my hand over the area [off the physical body] where she feared being hit again until I felt it dissolve. She never got headaches again.

The 'story' here is framed in a way that makes it very appropriate as a teaching tool. The tutor indicates that 'all sorts of treatments' had not been effective, because the real body-story – including the aetiology and the legacy of that in the tissues – had not been understood fully. When that subtle 'palpable feeling' was 'noticed', the treatment was clear, even though it was not conventionally osteopathic. Value is assigned to this correct recognition of the body-story and, perhaps obviously, the cessation of the headaches.

In homeopathy, there is a massive range of potentially relevant aspects of the patient's experience and not every aspect of body-talk can be covered in a consultation. Therefore, student-homeopaths must learn to be comfortable with the *uncertainty* inherent in their case-taking and *flexible* in their approach to treatment. They must find a close enough match between the patient's state and one of the homeopathic remedies they have learnt. As this extract from a lecture on the remedy *Arsenicum* shows, the *character* in the story is the remedy, which contrasts with the biomedical tendency to refer to patients by their diagnosis ('the hernia in room three'). The implications of categorising patients by remedies, rather than disease labels, means that there is an intermingling of the physical and emotional patterns as part of a process, or story, rather than as a snapshot:

> *Arsenicums* need to be in control. This helps them to allay fears. Their fears are particularly around health and they fear death to their very core. So they carefully plan their day, make lists, are neat and tidy so that they know where things are. They are fastidious, perfectionists, and very driven. As the *Arsenicum* picture *goes deeper* the fear *extends* to worrying about their family being 'got' as well. So the *Arsenicum* starts with fear, so they turn to perfectionism to control it, but this takes a lot of energy so if they begin to not have enough energy they can become compulsive, so get OCD [Obsessive Compulsive Disorder]. *Then* they get more fears about being invaded, *which turns* into a deep depression, and *eventually* to suicidal impulses. *At this point* they may turn to knives for self-harm, and they fear committing suicide and fear hurting others or killing others. *When they reach deep pathology* they start to crumble at all levels and maybe become a recluse. Also they can become anorexic *at this point*, because of their fear of food [*my emphases*].

The assessment of the patient, then, is not 'OCD', for example, or even 'worn-down and exhausted', but 'has become worn-down and exhausted in an *Arsenicum*-like process'.

The construction of the body-story and the effects of the remedy itself are inseparable in homeopathy. Tutors reported that while sometimes taking a remedy preceded awareness and transformation at any level: 'remedies are little bundles of awareness, little parachutes'; for another 'the healing moment was her acknowledgement [of her reasons for her fatigue] and the remedy supported that'. The student's reflexive capabilities are crucial to the success of this process: 'hold up a mirror [to the patient], do not take it [their stuff] on . . . if you can't be a mirror, [it] may be best to refer the person on. Be honest about who you are'. In this way the students' bodies and biographies are explicitly implicated as central to their ability to carry out their work.

Narrative and healing

As Hyden (1997) puts it 'the narrative is one of several cultural forms available to us for conveying, expressing or formulating our experience of illness and suffering' (1997: 64). The findings in this chapter extend the sociological literature on narrative and healing, particularly where empirical work that draws on practices with dualist conceptions of the mind and body underpins current theory. In particular, while much discussion in the medical sphere has begun to recognise the importance of narrative (*e.g.* Charon and Montello 2002, Greenhalgh and Hurwitz 1998), it usually is couched in terms that do not threaten the 'real business' of medical diagnosis and treatment, except insofar as it assists case management and concordance. Both the osteopaths and homeopaths learn that narratives are integral to both 'diagnosis' and the healing process itself. These different professional modes of narrative construction can destabilise Cartesian dualism and give attention in different ways to the 'body' and embodiment in the construction of narratives of coping and aetiology.

The impact of these different social relations of healthcare work can have a profound impact on the health and embodied experiences of patients. Baarts and Pederson (2009) observe that CAM clients, due to the repeated corporeal reflections that they make over time as a result of CAM treatment, form a 'coherent body narrative'. They draw on Leder's (1990) influential work on the 'absent' body, where he argues that undertaking daily habitual behaviours or being in a state of 'health' render the body invisible: it 'disappears'. By contrast, he argues that illness can cause the body to 'dys-appear': 'Insofar as the body seizes our awareness particularly at times of disturbance, it can come to appear "Other" and opposed to the self. Such experiences then play a part in buttressing Cartesian dualism' (Leder 1990: 70). Baarts and Pederson contend that CAM 'profoundly disrupts modes of bodily disappearance' (2009: 2) making clients more aware of their bodies and their embodiment even when they no longer suffer from pain or illness. However, probably as an artefact of their phenomenological approach and focus on patients, rather than the therapeutic interaction, their argument about narratives does not fundamentally challenge mind/body dualism. They conceptualise 'body talk' as the dialogue during CAM treatments and 'body work' as the CAM treatments themselves. These formulations retain an assumption of the primacy of mind over body, and this is underpinned by their use of the concept of 'bodily mastery' to describe the experiences of the clients.

Nonetheless, there are some important echoes of the existing literature on storytelling and narrative in illness in these data, such as the reasons patients need to voice illness narratives: they give sufferers of illness the chance to create a public voice for their experiences, to place the illness experience in the context of wider life experience and the opportunity to reinforce their own voice and experiences when confronted with the voice of biomedicine (Frank 1994). In the context of the cultural dominance of the biomedical model which often 'silences' the 'voice of the lifeworld' (Mishler 1990), it is particularly important for student CAM practitioners to learn skills that enable them to 'produce a patient that talks' (Gale 2008).

It is tempting to say that the 'body-stories' described in this chapter are closer to lay models of illness, but we should be careful not to fall into the trap of assuming that these narratives are more 'authentic'. While there is evidence to suggest that patients are likely to be more critical and sceptical of CAM approaches than they are of conventional medical practice (May and Sirur 1998), the models of health and healing that the homeopaths and osteopaths use are still likely to dominate the encounter. The practitioners, after all, have the expertise and develop the habit of constructing stories that 'fit' their own therapeutic model (Gale 2008). We could speculate that as the patient becomes more expert at this liminal state of reflexive embodiment, s/he may challenge the practitioner's interpretations. It is also possible that as the practitioner becomes more experienced, they may either be better able to cope with the uncertainty of practice and so more open to negotiation of the body-story or their practice may become habit driven and less reflexive (unless they undertake activities, such as CPD, mentoring or teaching others, that nurture this).

Body work and embodied work

This chapter provides empirical evidence to support the argument that 'body work occupations appear to be shaped, in the first place, by definitions of the body that guide or empower workers in relation to it' (Wolkowitz 2002: 500). The findings show that the kind of body-talk that is produced and listened to in osteopathy and homeopathy consultations is shaped by philosophical beliefs about health and the healing process. Emphases both on a 'body' that may be able to communicate more clearly than consciously-generated explanations and on 'embodiment' disrupts mind/body dualism. The concept of body-talk, which can be used to understand part of the work that happens in the consultation, is designed to highlight the agency of the embodied patient. This, thereby, challenges the inevitability of the taken-for-granted dualist notion that the central dynamic in the therapeutic encounter is the mind of the doctor working upon the body of the patient (and, hence, that the mind of the patient and the body of the doctor are not relevant).

Following on from this, not only is the embodiment of the student-practitioner relevant, it is explicitly valued at the Colleges of Homeopathy and Osteopathy. While we would recognise as ridiculous the suggestion that medical students could be expected to 'try out' medication or surgery on themselves, the osteopathy and homeopathy students are expected to experience 'being a patient' not only through continued treatment by a qualified practitioner but in the very fabric of the organisation of training which requires that the students explore their concepts of health and healing and practise their developing skills with each other. During this time the day-to-day absence of the lived body (Leder 1990) is made visible for the students as they experience new embodied sensations and develop new embodied knowledge. 'Playing' the roles of osteopath/homeopath and patient is fundamental to the development of a sense of intersubjectivity and an ability to be reflexive (Crossley 2001: 144). These new modes of embodied intersubjectivity mean that CAM practitioners are very literally and explicitly doing 'embodied work'. Doing 'work on yourself' is commonplace language in CAM communities and is required of both patients and practitioners for a successful therapeutic encounter.

The type of body work found in CAM could be located in the wider context of late modernity. Giddens (1991) for instance has noted the potential for reflexively monitored change amidst diverse choices in late modern society. Some commentators, in a similar vein, have argued that CAM fails to challenge the status quo because any changes are only at an individual level (Coward 1989). Others have noted that broader health movements, which stress 'wellness' and the 'sacred', are becoming increasingly important (Williams 2003). The data presented in this chapter certainly convey a sense of activism in the way the practitioners learn to challenge biomedical separation between mental/emotional and physical health and the divorce of medical practice from spiritual health, hence facilitating an alternative (non-biomedical) narrative to emerge. Praxis perhaps could have the potential to subvert the political order (in which biomedical, heterosexist, racist and sexist discourses dominate) because for the students 'the reconstruction of knowledge is inseparable from the reconstruction of the self' (Jaggar 1989: 164). In this way, practising body work could bring into being an alternative political identity and constitute a form of embodied activism (Scott 1997, 1998). Of course, if this is the 'ideal' then it is differentially realised in practice because it is limited by the practicalities of the learning environment (Gale 2008) or by the constraining cultural discourses and regulatory and governance systems which affect the ability to practise and run a successful and legally compliant business. The dominance of body/mind dualism and rationalism may be destabilised but it is not overturned.

Future research

As this book is a developmental introduction to the concept of body work, it seems apposite to talk some more about potential future agendas in relation to CAM that this chapter has begun to touch on. Wolkowitz (2002) calls for body work to be examined in terms of its social relations (divisions of labour and workplace interactions) as well as the definitions of the body that different practices draw on. More widely, this ties into research on 'new' forms of work that go beyond the traditional production/consumption binary and take place outside conventional employment structures (Pettinger et al. 2006).

The social characteristics of the CAM workforce remain unstudied. From anecdotal observations, the demographics of the student populations in my study and by scanning professional registers, it appears that many practitioners are women, often older, embarking on a second career or returning to work after having children. Increased regulation in osteopathy seems to have led to a reduction in the average age of students at the College of Osteopathy over the last 10 years. However, this area would bear more systematic study. It may be of interest to explore further the professional status of CAM practitioners through the lens of body work debates. Twigg (2000) argues that body work is 'ambivalent' because it verges on the taboo areas of sexuality and human waste. All body work, she argues, is 'potentially demeaning work and when undertaken by high status individuals it is typically accompanied by distancing techniques' (2000: 391), what she terms a 'dematerializing tendency'. Body work then is bound up with the division of labour that occurs usually along gendered and racialised lines (Wolkowitz 2002). CAM does not sit easily in this framework, perhaps because the 'silencing' of the body in care work can only be understood when located in a division of labour that is underpinned by mind/body dualism. Perhaps a body that is seen as an 'intelligent' agent does not have the same demeaning associations.

The nature of the social relations of CAM are also poorly understood. As many practitioners work independently there is much less scope for the 'outsourcing' of unpleasant or routine tasks to lower paid and lower status workers, although some busy practitioners do employ receptionists or cleaners. The patient's body is not divided up to fit a complex, socially-mediated and hierarchical division of labour. Moreover, access to the patient's body granted to orthodox health practitioners by their high social status and legal standing cannot be assumed in CAM practice. Access must be carefully negotiated with the recipient of the treatment, and the location of these therapies in the private sphere precludes the possibility of (legal) forced bodily contact or treatment, such as when people are sectioned. These characteristics may be related to the observation that CAM patients often feel that their healthcare is more personalised and holistic and that they have more control over the encounter (Sharma 1992). Further exploration of work relations in this field and its embodied implications for patients and practitioners would be useful.

Wolkowitz (2002) points out that how far the 'holism' espoused by CAM practitioners is 'actually realised in embodied interactions, rather than remaining at the level of discourse' may be 'influenced by conditions of employment, including the managerial philosophies, staffing policies and payment systems that have evolved in the context of custom and practice of different occupations' (2002: 503). There are increasing drives for more 'professionalism' in the CAM field and for 'integration' of systems with conventional medicine, although these developments are not universally supported by CAM professionals (Schneirov and Geczik 2002). These changes are altering the demographics of the practitioner population and the way in which CAM practice is regulated, which will have an impact on power relations in the embodied interactions in the therapeutic encounter. Research is clearly needed to understand how practitioners negotiate these regulatory frameworks, which would be able to extend sociological work on the links between the development of professions, gender and the dominance of biomedical discourses (Saks 2003, Stacey 1988, Witz 1992).

Conclusions

Listening to body-talk and constructing body-stories have been presented as aspects of body work in the context of CAM practice. Learning to *listen to body-talk* is a useful way to think about the different practical methods that students use to collect the relevant information that they need about the embodied patient. This is because body-talk as a concept allows us to explore the possibility that the embodied patient is not a passive recipient of healthcare, but that the 'body', as conceptualised in homeopathic and osteopathic theory, is able to communicate its distress and its needs. *Constructing body-stories* is central to the therapeutic encounter. Body-stories are, in both practices, co-produced through the embodied interaction between patient and practitioner, although the balance of power is not necessarily symmetrical in this interaction. The construction of the body-story is an important clinical task for the practitioner and one that is fundamental to the success of the treatment; the shape of the body-story, therefore, must be congruent with the concept of health and healing that the practitioner is using. For the osteopaths, it is central to building a dynamic and integrative model of the embodied patient. For the homeopaths, they must get enough detail about the body-story of their patient to be able to ascertain which remedy picture it is most similar to.

These data have enabled a critical examination of CAM as a form of body work. Understanding the narrative construction at the heart of the therapeutic encounter challenges biomedical and Cartesian notions of the primacy of mind over body. In the CAM model, both practitioner and patient play an important and intersubjective role in the embodied work because the model demands that the body of the patient is not only to be worked on, but is listened to (because it is capable of communicating in a number of ways). In addition, I have demonstrated that narrative construction is a core element of the model of healing in osteopathy and homeopathy, which contrasts with its role as a supplement to biomedical interventions. There has also been a discussion on the observation that body work is also embodied work and that practitioners are explicitly taught to reflexively monitor their practices. In summary, it is vital to recognise that different models of the 'body', particularly those that challenge mind/body dualism, can fundamentally shift both the nature and power relations of body work.

Acknowledgements

This research was funded by the Economic and Social Research Council, through their Postgraduate Studentship programme. Thanks are due to my supervisors, Professor Simon Williams and Dr Carol Wolkowitz, for their guidance, the anonymous reviewers and the editors of this volume for their helpful comments, and, last but not least, my participants, who welcomed me into their lives for a year and showed me their world.

Notes

1   It is important to be wary of caricaturing either biomedicine or CAM, especially in relation to the label of 'holism'. Boundaries between orthodox and alternative medicine are not as stable or impermeable as either scientists or practitioners from either 'side' have generally made them out to be (Cant, S. and Sharma, U. (1999), *A New Medical Pluralism?* London: UCL Press.) There is clearly diversity of practice under the banner of CAM, as there is a multiplicity of therapies, many of which have vastly different ontological, epistemological and cultural bases, and the biomedical model is also only an 'ideal type' representation of 'modern' or 'scientific' medicine. It is a foundation (conceptual not historical) for the day-to-day practice of those working in heterogeneous ways within the orthodox healthcare professions. General practitioners, in particular, often consider themselves to be 'holistic' in approach. I hope that the data presented will help draw out the distinctive approaches of the osteopaths and homeopaths in relation to 'holism' and the 'body'. See also Williams, S.J. (2003), *Medicine and the Body*, London, Sage, for a helpful discussion on different models of health and the body.

2   The House of Lords Select committee for Science and Technology produced a report on CAM in 2000 which identified five 'Professionally Organised Alternative Therapies'. These were osteopathy and chiropratic which are both now statutorily regulated, herbal medicine, acupuncture and homeopathy.

References

Baarts, C. and Pedersen, I.K. (2009) Derivative benefits: exploring the body through complementary and alternative medicine, *Sociology of Health and Illness*, 31, 5, 1–15.
Barrett, M. (2000) Sociology and the metaphorical tiger. In Gilroy, P., Grossberg, L. and McRobbie, A. (eds) *Without Guarantees; in Honour of Stuart Hall*. London: Verso.
Belenky, M.F., Clinchy, B.M., Goldberger, N.R. and Tarule, J.M. (1997) *Women's Ways of Knowing: the Development of Self, Voice and Mind* (2nd Edition). New York: Basic Books.
Bulmer, M. (1984) *The Chicago School of Sociology: Institutionalization, Diversity and the Rise of Sociological Research*. Chicago: University of Chicago Press.
Bury, M. (1982) Chronic illness as biographical disruption, *Sociology of Health and Illness*, 4, 2, 167–82.
Cant, S. and Sharma, U. (1999) *A New Medical Pluralism?* London: UCL Press.
Cassell, J. (1998) *The Woman in the Surgeon's Body*. London: Harvard University Press.
Charon, R. and Montello, M. (2002) *Stories Matter: the Role of Narrative in Medical Ethics*. London: Routledge.
Coward, R. (1989) *The Whole Truth: the Myth of Alternative Health*. London: Faber and Faber.
Crossley, N. (2001) *The Social Body: Habit, Identity and Desire*. London: Sage.

Frank, A. (1994) Reclaiming an ophan genre: the first person narrative of illness, *Literature and Medicine*, 13, 1–21.

Gale, N.K. (2008) Promoting patient-practitioner partnership in clinical training: a critical evaluation, *Learning in Health and Social Care*, 8, 1, 13–21.

Gale, N.K. (2010) The embodied ethnographer: journeys in a healthcare sub-culture, *International Journal of Qualitative Methods*, 9, 2, 206–223.

Geertz, C. (1973) *The Interpretation of Cultures*. London: Fontana Press.

Giddens, A. (1991) *Modernity and Self-Identity: Self and Society in the Late Modern Age*. Stanford: Stanford University Press.

Gimlin, D. (2007) What is 'body work'? A review of the literature, *Sociology Compass*, 1, 1, 353–70.

Greenhalgh, T. and Hurwitz, B. (eds) (1998) *Narrative Based Medicine: Dialogue and Discourse in Clinical Practice*. London: BMJ Books.

Jaggar, A.M. (1989) Love and knowledge: emotion in feminist epistemology. In Jaggar, A.M. and Bordo, S.R. (eds) *Gender/Body/Knowledge: Feminist Reconstructions of Being and Knowing*. London: Routledge.

Kuhn, T.S. (1962) *The Structure of Scientific Revolutions*. London: University of Chicago Press.

Lawler, J. (1991) *Behind the Screens: Nursing, Somology and the Problem of the Body*. London: Churchill Livingstone.

Leder, D. (1990) *The Absent Body*. London: University of Chicago Press.

Malinowski, B. (1922) *Argonauts of the Western Pacific: an Account of Native Enterprise and Adventure in the Archipelagos of Melanesian New Guinea*. London: Routledge and Kegan Paul.

May, C. and Sirur, D. (1998) Art, science and placebo: incorporating homeopathy in general practice, *Sociology of Health and Illness*, 20, 2, 168–90.

McKone, W.L. (2001) *Osteopathic Medicine: Philosophy, Principles and Practice*. Oxford: Blackwell Science.

Mishler, E.G. (1990) The struggle between the voice of medicine and the voice of the lifeworld. in Conrad, P. and Kern, R. (eds) *The Sociology of Health and Illness: Critical Perspectives* (3rd Edition). New York: St Martins Press.

Pettinger, L., Parry, J., Taylor, R. and Glucksmann, M. (2005) *A new sociology of work? Sociological Review monographs*. Oxford: Blackwell.

Saks, M. (2003) *Orthodox and Alternative Medicine: Politics, Professionalization and Health Care*. London: Sage.

Schneirov, M. and Geczik, J.D. (2002) Alternative health and the challenges of institutionalization, *Health: an Interdisciplinary Journal for the Social Study of Health, Illness and Medicine*, 6, 201.

Scott, A. (1997) The knowledge in our bones: standpoint theory, alternative health and the quantum model of the body. In Maynard, M. (ed.) *Science and the Construction of Women*. London: UCL Press.

Scott, A. (1998) Homoeopathy as a feminist form of medicine, *Sociology of Health and Illness*, 20, 2, 191–214.

Sharma, U. (1992) *Complementary Medicine Today: Practitioners and Patients*. London: Routledge.

Stacey, M. (1988) *The Sociology of Health and Healing*. London: Routledge.

Twigg, J. (2000) Carework as a form of bodywork, *Ageing and Society*, 20, 389–411.

Williams, S.J. (2003) *Medicine and the Body*. London: Sage.

Williams, S.J. and Bendelow, G. (1998) *The Lived Body: Sociological Themes, Embodied Issues*. London: Routledge.

Witz, A. (1992) *Professions and Patriarchy*. London: Routledge.

Wolkowitz, C. (2002) The social relations of body work, *Work, Employment and Society*, 16, 3, 497–510.

Wolkowitz, C. (2006) *Bodies at Work*. London: Sage.

6

Educating with the hands: working on the body/self in Alexander Technique
Jennifer Tarr

Introduction

In August 2008, the *British Medical Journal* (BMJ), published the results of a randomised controlled trial indicating that lessons in the Alexander Technique had long-term benefits for back pain patients, and are more effective than prescriptions for either massage or exercise (Little *et al.* 2008). A total of 579 UK patients with back pain were randomly assigned to three control groups, giving this study the large-scale body of data needed to be taken seriously by the medical community. Given the difficulties that treating back pain offers for biomedicine (Tait and Chinball 1997, Rhodes *et al.* 1999), the study results looked promising for the more widespread adoption of the Alexander Technique. While the Technique is often classified broadly as a complementary therapy and as such has received little scientific and medical attention in terms of its efficacy, its founder F.M. Alexander had always intended his work to be taken up by the medical profession. His final book, *The Universal Constant in Living*, makes particular attempts to relate his work to biomedicine, noting:

> Ever since I first started taking pupils, medical men have been sending me their patients because they believed that I had evolved a sound technique. I am deeply indebted to them for their encouragement and support, and especially for the effort they are now making to bring a knowledge of my technique to the notice of those who are responsible for determining the range and nature of the medical curriculum with the aim of its being included in medical training. (Alexander 2000 [1941]: 13)

This is not the first time Alexander Technique has appeared in the BMJ; a review of Alexander's second book, *Constructive Conscious Control of the Individual*, was published by the BMJ in May 1924 and concluded that the Technique 'would certainly appear to have something of value to communicate to the medical profession' (in Alexander 2000 [1941]: 13). In 1937, 19 doctors wrote a letter to the BMJ supporting further investigation of the Technique from a medical perspective (Fischer 2008: 1502).

Yet the relationship between Alexander Technique and mainstream healthcare remains an ambivalent one. Using data from an ethnographic study incorporating participant observation, semi-structured interviewing, and textual analysis of documents, this chapter

Body Work in Health and Social Care, First Edition. Edited by Julia Twigg, Carol Wolkowitz, Rachel Lara Cohen and Sarah Nettleton.

examines the tensions between biomedicine and the Technique. It argues that while the Alexander Technique may have much to offer as a physical practice, the discursive strategies in which it is framed, specifically its overreliance on its founder and on a particular view of nature and evolution, as well as its view of the self, make it unlikely to receive mainstream medical acceptance. In making a distinction between embodied practice and discourse, Crossley's (1994, 1996) argument that discourse and embodiment are two sides of the same coin is followed, and that one need not choose between the two. Against approaches from sociology of the body which have taken up a 'corporeal realist' approach (Shilling 2004), as a way of combining these two themes, I would argue that in some circumstances, examining discourses and embodiment in contrast rather than attempting to resolve the tensions between them can provide productive insights.

While clearly a form of body work in the sense that it 'takes the body as its immediate site of labour, involving intimate, messy contact with the (frequently supine or naked) body, its orifices or products through touch or close proximity' (Wolkowitz 2002: 497), the Technique goes out of its way to avoid addressing the body as such. By positioning itself as holistic in the sense that it works on the integrated body and mind, it strives to overcome mind-body dualism by addressing the self, as phrases such as 'good use of the self' attest. This distancing from the body has a twofold effect: it both emphasises the conscious nature of the work which lies at its core, and also detaches it from a concern with the negative aspects of the body for which body work is stigmatised, such as its relation to sexuality, waste products, and decline (Twigg 2000).

The Alexander Technique is often categorised as a form of complementary and alternative medicine (CAM), although this relationship is somewhat ambivalent. Coward (1989) includes the Alexander Technique in her study of alternative health because it shares similar ideas, such as an emphasis on one founding figure and on being 'natural'. Sharma (1992: 4), on the other hand, excludes the Alexander Technique from her own study of CAM because it does not purport to cure disease, but only to re-educate people to use their bodies more efficiently. For her, the defining characteristics of complementary or alternative medicine are that it claims to be curative, has some body of knowledge or theory about health and illness, and requires some kind of expert intervention on the part of a practitioner (1992: 4). Here, this study takes the position that although it is not curative or a form of medicine as such, the Technique shares some characteristics with CAM as a health practice operating outside mainstream health and social care, making research in this area relevant to it.

The chapter begins by describing the Alexander Technique and outlining the aims and scope of the study on which this chapter was based. It goes on to describe the embodied practice of the Technique, and then contrast this with the discourses in which it is embedded as a 'technique of the self' (Foucault 1985, 1986), through examining the authorities or modes of subjection it uses to justify what it does, how its aims and aspirations of holism ally it more closely with CAM than with biomedicine, and how its notion of the self as the substance to be worked upon both distances the work from the negative connotations of body work and also creates a tension between the Technique and mainstream healthcare practices which concern themselves with the body.

What is the Alexander Technique?

The Alexander Technique is a form of body work which seeks to educate its pupils to use their bodies more efficiently in everyday movement. It is usually taught in one-to-one sessions between a teacher and pupil, which last between half an hour and 45 minutes. These sessions include activities to make pupils aware that they suffer from what the Technique calls 'faulty sensory awareness' and to enable them to differentiate aspects of their movement and thereby develop more precise awareness of their bodily use. Lessons often include activities such as standing and sitting from a chair, and are generally concluded with 'table work' where, in common with body work practices such as massage, pupils lie on the table and their bodies are passively manipulated by the teacher.

The Technique was developed in the late 19th century by Frederick Matthias Alexander, a Tasmanian actor and elocutionist who began to lose his voice while reciting, and developed his own method for overcoming this difficulty (Alexander 1985 [1932]). He moved to London in 1904 to promote his work and later set up a teacher training programme in the neighbourhood of Holland Park. He died in 1955 and his work is continued by thousands of Alexander Technique teachers worldwide (STAT 2009).

Even as it has sought medical recognition in order to legitimise itself, the Alexander Technique has held biomedicine at arm's length since its inception. Alexander's story of founding the Technique describes how he lost his voice during recitations. His physician prescribed rest, which initially made the problem recede, but as soon as he returned to elocution he began to have difficulties again. At this point he recounts making the decision to pursue his own means for correcting the problem. He did this through regular self-observation in the mirror while he was reciting, which led him to the discovery that he was throwing his head back as he spoke, thereby restricting his vocal chords. While this use 'felt natural' to him, such a feeling was ultimately untrustworthy and led him into error (Alexander 1985 [1932]: 21). The key process of the Alexander Technique is the inhibition of the initial desire to react to a particular stimulus, in order to consider and apply conscious control to the response. Alexander notes that when he had cured his tendency to revert to wrong use in reciting, it also improved throat and vocal trouble and respiratory difficulties he had suffered since birth (Alexander 1985 [1932]: 36). While Staring (1996, 1997) has cast doubt on the authenticity of Alexander's tale of individual triumph in the face of medical bafflement about his condition, it remains prevalent, serving the function of establishing Alexander's authority as someone with unique knowledge of the body/self not found in biomedical practice.

Study design

The data analysed here emerge from a larger study of a range of somatic education techniques. The research methods included participant observation, analysis of the texts written by the founders of these techniques, and 28 semi-structured interviews undertaken with professional practitioners and pupils. The majority of interviews (17) were conducted with Alexander Technique teachers and pupils. The study aimed to examine how the discourses put forward by the founders of these techniques were adapted by contemporary practitioners and whether and how these discourses related to their embodied practices.

The texts analysed in this study included Alexander's four books, *Man's Supreme Inheritance* (1910); *Constructive Conscious Control of the Individual* (1923); *The Use of the Self* (1932); *The Universal Constant in Living* (1941). They were analysed using a Foucauldian approach, examining key discourses of these techniques as 'techniques of the self' (Foucault 1985, 1986). Foucault notes that techniques of the self are 'intentional and voluntary actions, by which men not only set themselves rules of conduct, but also seek to transform themselves, to change themselves in their singular being, and to make their life into an *oeuvre* that carries certain aesthetic values and meets certain stylistic criteria' (1985: 10–11). While the Alexander Technique clearly meets this definition, biomedicine is not here contrasted as a 'technique of the self' as such, since much medical practice lacks these transformative ethical/aesthetic dimensions.

I undertook participant observation in Alexander Technique lessons on a regular basis for a period of approximately 18 months. During this time, I had 30 lessons with one Alexander teacher who played the role of 'key informant' in this study. These lessons were tape recorded and reconstructed in fieldnotes. Alexander Technique participants were recruited for interviews primarily through snowball sampling strategies, as well as advertisements in training centres and an e-mail sent to the Society of Teachers of the Alexander Technique (STAT) list. Ten male and seven female participants were interviewed; nine were teachers and eight were pupils. Their ages ranged from 20 to 70 with most in their thirties and forties. The range of experience was broad, from a pupil who had three months of lessons to a teacher who had practised for over 30 years. On average, pupils tended to have had two to three years' experience with the Technique while teachers' experience averaged around ten years. Participants were predominantly white European, including English, Scottish, Finnish, Danish, Swiss, and Dutch, although three were of Indian, Japanese, or Chinese ancestry. Interview data were entered into NVivo and analysed using a qualitative thematic approach, using themes drawn from the interview questions, participant observation and the analysis of texts.

Participants were based in a major urban centre, where the number of Alexander Technique practitioners means that opportunities for interacting with other practitioners as well as competition for pupils are much greater. Teachers were largely recruited via e-mail and therefore access was limited to those who regularly used this medium. Participant observation was undertaken with full overt disclosure of the purposes of the research. A letter explaining the research was provided and the author's Alexander teacher agreed to participate and to allow to the recording and transcribing of lessons for later publication. He read and verified the account of the lessons. Interview participants were told the purpose of the research and advised that they could refuse to answer any questions and withdraw from the research or terminate the interview at any time without consequence to themselves. Pseudonyms are used throughout the text and identifying details have been obscured.

Knowledge in the hands

As a form of body work, the Alexander Technique is what Merleau-Ponty referred to as 'knowledge in the hands' (1962: 144). For Merleau-Ponty, all habit is a kind of embodied knowledge, neither controlled by conscious reflection nor merely a matter of blind physiological response to a stimulus. However, Shusterman (2004) observes that Merleau-Ponty's notion of habit is a limited one because he accounts only for unconscious bodily awareness, in an effort to defend tacit knowledge and because he believed that conscious awareness could also inhibit both our perceptions of such knowledge and the efficiency with which it functioned. Shusterman suggests a revised understanding of the consciousness of habit which includes four levels of awareness: first, that of the unconscious awareness which occurs in sleep; second, conscious perception without explicit awareness, such as the ability to navigate a doorframe without being aware of its dimensions; third, conscious awareness with explicit perception, where, for example, one is aware of being short of breath; and finally self-conscious awareness with explicit perception, where one is aware of what the Alexander Technique would call the 'means-whereby' one undertakes an action, so, for example, not only of being short of breath but of the way in which one is breathing (Shusterman 2004: 158).

He goes on to argue that methods such as the Alexander Technique bring awareness to the latter two levels. He argues that the level of unreflected habit championed by Merleau-Ponty is insufficient because we can acquire bad habits as easily as good ones, and habitual behaviours cannot correct these since they are precisely what are wrong. Somatic techniques such as the Alexander Technique, effect this improvement by bringing unconscious habit to conscious critical reflection so that it can be worked on (2004: 165).[1]

Using Shusterman's revision of Merleau-Ponty's phenomenology, we can begin to understand how the Alexander Technique works as an embodied practice. The Technique is transmitted through the hands of the Alexander teacher, whose manual adjustments of the pupil convey the sense of the work and how the body/self is to be aligned. Conscious control is an important part of this: the pupil is asked to inhibit, or to 'not react' to a particular stimulus. In *The Use of the Self*, Alexander described the process fundamental to his work: first, initial responses to a stimulus must be inhibited; second, the directions for 'primary control' of the head-neck-back relationship should be projected until sufficiently well absorbed to respond to the stimulus; third, while still projecting these directions for new use, a fresh decision should be made about whether or not to respond to the stimulus; and finally some kind of response to it should be undertaken (Alexander 1985 [1932]: 33–4). One of the most common stimuli provided in lessons is a chair, and pupils are asked to practise standing and sitting without collapsing the proper alignment of the head-neck-back relationship, sometimes referred to as the 'central core'. When asked to stand up from a chair, most people shorten their necks and look up, throwing their backs into poor alignment. With the Alexander Technique, the head and neck are directed to go 'forward and up', and they lead the action of the body.

In one lesson, my Alexander teacher began to show me how he went about working on a pupil. He placed my arms in a rounded position in front of me and then stood in between them so my hands were on his chest and back. 'From that place you can direct yourself up. Keep dropping your shoulders but keep thinking about sending your head forward and up. You're not interested in how to direct my body, you're interested in how to stay back, so you can see more of the reaction clearly'. He then said his temptation was to 'end-gain', as a teacher, by collapsing his head-neck-back relationship, but indicated that he had to focus on his own relationship and on 'non-doing' rather than focusing on my use. Good use of one's self while teaching is therefore at least as important as the activities undertaken.

Among teachers of the Alexander Technique, proximity to Alexander and/or the teachers he trained is considered a mark of distinction. A teacher who trained with someone who was taught directly by Alexander has higher status than someone who is more removed from him. This is not simply because the former are likely to have more years of experience, but also because the work is seen as most authentic at its source. This is not only the idolisation of the founder which occurs in many forms of complementary and alternative health (Coward 1989: 36). It is also that the work is transmitted physically, and it is only through physical work on the body that it can be understood. If Alexander's hands are believed to have held unique skills, then access to others who have been worked on by him – that is, to whom the work has been transmitted through his hands – is a way of accessing higher quality work. This, however, ignores the ways in which the Technique has developed since Alexander's time, and the possibility that very experienced teachers may have skills as good or even better than those of Alexander himself. For instance, sedimented years of experience with a variety of teachers might lead to a wider range of skills and abilities in transmitting the Technique to others.

The day I spent at a teacher training school was a clear indicator of the extent to which experience matters. Alexander teachers train for three hours per day, every weekday for 30 weeks a year over three years. Largely, this training is conducted through hands-on experience, although it will also include discussion and reading from Alexander's books or other relevant texts. On the morning when I visited, a circle of chairs was arranged in the living room of a private home, and the students, about 10 in total, were gradually rising and sitting from them, focusing on inhibiting their initial reactions, and projecting directions for good use of the self. They continued this for over an hour, while the two teachers circulated and worked on each student in turn for between 5 and 15 minutes. Toward the end of this session, two more experienced students approached with their teacher's encouragement and asked if they could work on me. They guided me in sitting and standing from the chair, but I found their hands uncertain and their touch hesitant. This made it difficult for me to follow the directions they were attempting to convey. Both they and I came away frustrated by the experience. Both trainees were relatively advanced within the training programme, which indicates the degree of skill required to embody and teach the Alexander Technique. This experience contrasted strongly with one later in the day, where one of the teachers running the training course did some work on me as part of a lesson to his pupils. He had over 40 years of experience, and I was struck by the certainty conveyed through his hands, which immediately enabled me to use my legs in a new way while sitting down into the chair. While his touch was not excessive, he was able to transmit the work to me using relatively few adjustments of my head and neck and clear, straightforward verbal directions. His experience of teaching and his ability to embody the work were a result of his years of practice at teaching and transmitting the work through refining his own use of himself.

Nature and evolution in the Alexander Technique

The embodied practices of the Alexander Technique are only one aspect of the work. There is also the question of what Alexander teachers believe the Technique does, and what they take as authoritative about it. Foucault's analytic framework for 'techniques of the self' can usefully shed light on the discourses at work within the Alexander Technique. Foucault identifies four characteristics common to all techniques of the self (1985: 26–7): they contain forms of ethical work or techniques to be practised, an ethical substance or way in which the subject relates to him or herself, modes of subjection or authorities who are appealed to for validation, and a telos, or objectives and aspirations behind these practices. Looking at the Alexander Technique through this lens, it becomes possible to see why the Technique is incompatible with biomedicine in a way that is not apparent from its practices.

The physical practices of the Technique form the ethical work it does, because work on the body is also seen as work on the self. The self is the 'ethical substance' upon which it works; through the attainment of conscious control and consideration of the 'means-whereby' an activity is achieved, rather than 'end-gaining' by undertaking the activity using old, habitual patterns of use. The telos behind the Alexander Technique is body/self awareness. The increased awareness gained by the application of conscious control is one which was to lead humanity to regain what Alexander saw as a natural evolutionary inheritance. Nature and evolution form the modes of subjection in the Alexander Technique, as interpreted by Alexander himself. It is within these modes of subjection that the most striking incompatibilities with biomedicine are to be found.

Alexander believed humanity was physically degenerating, a belief he drew from the discourses of physical culture and eugenics prevalent in the early part of the 20th century

(Searle 1976). His first two books set out his argument along these lines. In earlier times, he believed, human instinct had been sufficient to keep up with the demands of the environment, but as civilisation advanced, conscious control of the self had not kept pace. He wrote:

> In order to meet satisfactorily the new demands of civilisation, *it was essential that man should acquire a new way of directing and controlling the mechanisms of the psycho-physical organism as a whole*, mechanisms which in the savage state had been kept up, of necessity, to a high standard of co-ordination by their use in securing the creature's daily food and in meeting the great 'physical' demands of this mode of life. (1987 [1923]: 5, italics in original)

In his earlier work, he made explicit links between his Technique and the eugenics movement (Alexander 1910), particularly in terms of the care and training of children in order to promote 'the science of race culture'. There is not space to explore this in detail here, but it is important to note that eugenics was a highly prevalent cultural discourse at that time and therefore his use of it is not unusual. He believed in an evolutionary scale on which some humans (namely children and 'savage' or non-Western peoples) were less developed and closer to animals and the state of nature (see also Jahoda 1999). The next stage of human evolution, he believed, required the application of constant conscious control to everyday movement and the use of the self, in order for humanity to stave off degeneration, and meet its full potential. While this was in no way a return to a state of nature, it was nonetheless, he argued, about regaining something which had been lost:

> *Re-education is not a process of adding something, but of restoring something.* It was to meet the need of restoring actual conditions of use and functioning which had been previously experienced and afterwards lost that my technique for the re-education of the use of the self was evolved (Alexander 2000 [1941]: 144–5, italics in original).

Such views about nature and evolution are not confined to Alexander's written texts. They also appear in some, although not all, of the discussions of Alexander teachers. In interviews, participants were asked whether they saw the Technique as 'natural', and what that might mean. Many participants took the view that the Technique was restoring a natural state, where 'natural' referred to a state prior to civilisation.[2] Several made comments which seemed straight out of Alexander's books:

> The technique is a kind of re-education, so the implication there is that we have this in us, we have this co-ordination in us. And of course you see it in kids, in very young children, that they have amazing posture and balance and with every movement the head leads and the body follows and all the things you learn in the Alexander Technique. It's quite frustrating to see that the little toddler has all that and more, and can squat for ages, or sit comfortably in any position with the spine really straight and the head sitting lightly on top of the spine and so on. So I think it's in us all to have that, it's like we have to peel away the layers of more problematic stuff that we've put on top of that for whatever reasons (Michael).

Two teachers more problematically echoed Alexander's views on race and culture as well; as one put it, 'there's always examples of people or cultures that have good use, but they're very few and far between, mainly people who live really away from Western life, more tribal sort of life, maybe Southern America, maybe some African tribes, maybe, I don't know, remote Chinese, Japanese ones'. These discourses are not the rule among Alexander teachers, but they do persist as an echo of Alexander's own views of some cultures as less 'civilised' than others.

Nature and evolution thus function as modes of subjection, or authorities, to which the Technique appeals to justify its practices. Alexander himself is presented as having unique insight into these practices; Coward (1989) notes of alternative therapies more generally that there is often 'a push to establish the therapy as deriving from a founding master, usually in the previous century. These founding figures then acquire . . . the status of one who understands and interprets natural truths' (Coward 1989: 36). The critical role played by Alexander as a founding figure further justifies the importance teachers place on lineage in teacher training.

Being unwilling to let go of the authority of Alexander and his discourses of nature and evolution, where proper order will be restored through the application of conscious control to the self, inhibits the Technique's more mainstream adoption. Further, while the Technique may be 'natural' in the sense that it does not involve chemical or surgical intervention on the body, it is nonetheless a culturally situated technique which draws heavily on the historical discourses of its time for its self-justification.

Complementary or alternative? Healthcare and the Alexander Technique

The allegiance to 'nature' rather than scientific research is one which aligns the Alexander Technique with CAM rather than with biomedicine (Coward 1989). It is also a key aspect of the telos behind the Alexander Technique, which aspires, through teaching conscious control of the self, to reclaim humanity's place within an evolutionary framework which Alexander believed had been lost. Where biomedicine treats the body as a series of parts and aspires to cure illness by identifying physiological problems and correcting them (Foucault 1973), the Alexander Technique aims at a holistic body/self awareness and use, which in turn is thought to have individual and social benefits. While this is a point of tension, it is not necessarily a contradiction; as Sharma points out, the reasons people use complementary and alternative health practices are not always because of a wholesale purchase of the philosophies behind them. Rather, 'most patients are simply using complementary medicine as a way of dealing with an intractable condition which orthodox medicine cannot cure to their satisfaction' (1992: 87).

In interviews, participants were asked about the relationship between the Alexander Technique, biomedicine and healthcare. In the responses, there was a clear division between patients and practitioners, particularly those teachers who had been involved with the Technique for some time. Pupils tended to be attracted to its 'alternative' status, and to see it as squarely outside mainstream healthcare because it addresses the whole person. Of the eight pupils interviewed, none seemed to hold biomedical practice in high esteem. Many had suffered an injury or illness which the medical profession had failed to adequately diagnose or treat. In some cases, this was what had led them to the Alexander Technique, as with one pupil and two teachers who suffered chronic pain while playing the violin which had drawn them to the work. As one pupil described, in relation to her disillusionment with biomedicine:

> We've gotten too clever for ourselves haven't we? We love mapping out things and deciphering things and this is caused by this, and what we're doing is that we're separating everything, and we rejoice greatly in mapping out those things and

diagnosing things, but sometimes I think the diagnosis becomes the aim rather than the cure. So we'll rejoice in saying, 'yes it's this that's wrong!' Great, now what? 'Eat some pills', you know, wonderful (Ingrid).

On the other hand, teachers tended to stress the potential positive relationship between the Technique and healthcare, and to emphasise its complementary nature. Saks notes that 'those practitioners most willing to adopt the term "complementary" rather than "alternative" medicine are those most likely to have political/ideological reasons for co-operating with medicine' (1994: 90), and greater co-operation with medicine would certainly serve the Alexander Technique well in terms of increasing its profile and attracting more pupils. As discussed previously, the desire for biomedical approval goes back to Alexander's own work, yet so does the ambivalence towards medicine, as exhibited in Alexander's description of his reasons for founding the Technique. When asked about the relationship with biomedicine, one senior teacher remarked:

I think it goes very well in terms of education. And I think it is going to be seen [as] health education. And I think the doctors and consultants who actually know about the Technique tend to approve of it. I think there's a problem with the NHS because the Technique is open-ended and relatively, in terms of education, it wouldn't be expensive, but in terms of treatment, it would be regarded as expensive . . . until there actually is the health service offering to patients the concept of health education, as part of the NHS, then it shouldn't be [covered under the NHS] because otherwise it tends to get regarded as treatment (Anthony).

The possibility of the Technique as health education was remarked upon by other teachers as well; several shared the position that while it would in theory be highly compatible with biomedicine, the contemporary focus of biomedical practice on treatment rather than prevention made this untenable. Other teachers stressed ways in which science was making discoveries in line with the Alexander Technique, for example in relation to the nervous system and neuromuscular patterning. One interviewee had been a practising medical specialist for several years, and talked about the difficulty of combining his previous medical career with his new work as an Alexander teacher:

It's a very political issue. I'm very comfortable giving Alexander lessons as an Alexander teacher in an Alexander centre. But if I do it as a treatment for the patients in hospitals, probably I'd find it a little bit difficult to give lessons because my attitude is going to change and it's like I have to give, you know. I mean the people's relationship is going to be quite different. Especially if I say I'm a [specialist] and giving the Alexander lessons . . . I don't want to bother to persuade medics to use this technique, they've too much work, so I don't bother. I'm quite comfortable being an Alexander teacher (Hiroshi).

Not surprisingly, when asked about the relationship to complementary and alternative medicine (CAM), patients and teachers tended to fall along the same lines. Patients were willing to see the work as alternative, while teachers were often more hesitant about the relationship to CAM. However, whether or not it fits within the category of complementary and alternative medicine, it certainly shares some characteristics with the work of practitioners in other forms of body work in this area: namely the importance of a founding figure as a key interpreter of 'nature', and a commitment to mind-body holism. In these, its telos is closer to that of CAM than to mainstream healthcare. While this is not necessarily an incommensurable tension given the pragmatic way many patients use CAM treatments, it may create further barriers to integration of the Technique with biomedicine.

The self as ethical substance

Another tension between biomedicine and the Alexander Technique is in what Foucault would call the 'ethical substance' upon which they work: while biomedicine works on the body, abstracted from the person, the Alexander Technique works on the self. The self to which Foucault refers in his concept of 'techniques of the self' often involves bodily or physical disciplines and not simply intellectual pursuits. The self addressed in the Alexander Technique is an integrated body/self, and the relationship between body and mind in the Technique is a complicated one.[3] While the Technique often frames itself as holistic and Alexander explicitly uses the word self in order to overcome mind/body dualism, the emphasis on conscious control is one which risks undermining this by reinscribing dualism as the conscious mind's control over the unruly, uneducated body. While both mind and body are involved in the Alexander Technique, mind would seem to have priority. However, as argued elsewhere (Tarr 2008: 496), proper alignment of the head-neck-back relationship is referred to as 'good use of the self,' making some part of the physical self (rather than a mental abstraction) the locus of selfhood. In this sense, the Technique is 'holistic'.

Yet there is a dual function in the use of the word self to describe the ethical substance being worked upon in the Alexander Technique. It also enables a distancing from any unpleasant connotations around the body and body work. Oerton and Phoenix (2001) have noted that the discourses of therapeutic massage practitioners and those of professional sex workers are parallel in the sense that for both, talk about the body is sublimated. For massage practitioners in particular, massage is desexualised by the way they speak of 'their work on and with bodies as having little to do with corporeality. Their narratives largely present touch as abstract and esoteric . . .' (Oerton and Phoenix 2001: 399). In these discourses, 'bodies are denuded of the body' (Oerton and Phoenix 2001: 400). By avoiding mention of the body itself, Alexander and his followers not only avoid mind/body dualism but also the negative associations of the body with sexuality. Encounters of Alexander Teachers and students are thereby framed in a way which is clearly professional, if somewhat abstracted from the actual embodied practices, which do unequivocally involve bodies. Teacher trainees are also not taught about the body in their training, as they get little in the way of anatomy or physiology grounding. Rather, as described above, their training is experiential and they read the texts of Alexander as background. It is Alexander's discourses, then, that they tend to reproduce in framing their work.

This tendency to avoid talking about bodies is apparent from the author's fieldnotes in both observations and the comments of the Alexander teacher. Body parts are referred to, but references to the body as a whole are less common. Moreover, they tend to take an abstracted rather than personal form: 'the' body rather than 'my/your' body. While mentions of bodies are more common in interviews and in lessons than they are in Alexander's writings, this abstraction is still prevalent. It serves a depersonalising function in what is ultimately quite intimate and personal work. As in other forms of body work (Oerton and Phoenix 2001, Twigg 2004: 393) there are restrictions on which areas of the body are touched: head, neck, back and arms are touched often, while legs are less commonly touched, and areas around the genitals are strictly off limits. This regulation and self-policing ensures that the work never crosses over into areas deemed inappropriate.

Like most body work outside mainstream health and social care, the Alexander Technique can afford to be selective about which parts of the body it addresses and why. Processes of waste and decay are rarely touched on in this work, and the relationships developed between pupil and teacher are not ones of dependence, but of education. This relationship is easier to sustain as egalitarian precisely because, as Wolkowitz points out, like most alternative practitioners Alexander teachers generally deal with whole, healthy, and continent bodies (2002: 505). In this their work differs from routine nursing or carework, with the consequence that Alexander teachers can perhaps more easily leave discourses on the body behind and subsume them in those of the self. As such, the self as ethical substance forms another point of discord between biomedical practices and the Alexander Technique.

Conclusion

In his analysis of techniques of the self, Foucault seeks to understand how individuals come to regulate themselves in line with particular norms, shaping themselves as ethical subjects. While biomedicine is also a way of regulating individuals in keeping with ethical norms, it has traditionally put less emphasis on ethical *self*-formation than on the power of the physician and the scientific apparatus – although the range of related self-health practices such as dietary advice and exercise regimes which have supported it certainly do become components of ethical self-fashioning. The key incompatibilities between the Alexander Technique and biomedicine are therefore embedded in their discursive frameworks, both in terms of the Technique's discourses about nature and evolution and tendency to treat Alexander as an authority figure and interpreter of these, and its emphasis on the self as a substance to be worked on which is not understood in physiological or anatomical terms. The purpose of this chapter has not been to critique either biomedicine or Alexander Technique as such, but rather to suggest reasons why straightforward incorporation of the Technique may have proven problematic.

Yet many of the discourses of the Alexander Technique are not necessary, practically speaking, for the Technique to be effective. Its embodied practices, whether or not they are read as a form of ethical work, seem to be beneficial. While Alexander teachers recommend courses of up to 30 lessons, the BMJ study suggested that six lessons, when followed by a prescription for exercise, were approximately 72 per cent as effective as 24 lessons and also retained their effectiveness after one year (Little *et al.* 2008). Greater involvement with biomedicine might in fact help Alexander teachers refine the claims they make for their work. Further, embodied practice can itself form a critique of Alexander's discourses about evolution and nature, since the Alexander Technique is clearly a social practice embedded in a particular set of historical and cultural knowledge claims.

While the Alexander Technique is a promising form of body work with potentially significant benefits for mainstream healthcare as a form of supplementary health education, the discursive knowledge systems in which it is embedded make it resistant to easy incorporation by biomedicine. If Alexander teachers want their work to be more widely recognised and appreciated, they would need to reframe it in terms which put less emphasis on Alexander as an authority figure and greater emphasis on physiological structures and processes, particularly during training. However, this may also serve to undermine the embodied knowledge which Alexander teachers possess, by shifting the focus of their learning toward biomedical and scientific knowledge frameworks and away from the less articulable forms of 'knowledge in the hands' which they practise. Whether Alexander teachers are willing and able to let go of Alexander and his evolutionary framework, and whether biomedicine and healthcare would then be more open to its practices, remains an open question.

Acknowledgements

The author would like to thank Universities UK for the Overseas Research Student Award which supported this research, the participants who gave generously of their time to take part in the project, and Helen Thomas for her insights. Thanks also to the anonymous reviewers whose feedback was extremely helpful in revising the manuscript.

Notes

1   Shusterman (2008), elsewhere critically considers Foucault's work in light of his own project of somaesthetics, although his attempt to refigure Foucault is not relevant to the purpose of the present study, which does not seek to make Foucault's work compatible with Alexander Technique's aims and objectives but only to examine how the Technique functions using Foucault's analytic framework of ethical self-fashioning.
2   The sense of the natural as precivilised, exemplified in the equation between children, non-Western peoples, and animals, is well explored in a number of texts including Wiber (1998) and Jahoda (1999).
3   Unfortunately there is not space here to further explore the similarities and differences between Foucault's and Alexander's use of the term self.

References

Alexander, F.M. (1910) *Man's Supreme Inheritance*. London: Methuen.
Alexander, F.M. (1985 [1932]) *The Use of the Self: Its Conscious Direction in Relation to Diagnosis, Functioning and the Control of Reaction*. London: Victor Gollancz Ltd.
Alexander, F.M. (1987 [1923]) *Constructive Conscious Control of the Individual*. London: Chaterson.
Alexander, F.M. (2000 [1941]) *The Universal Constant in Living*. London: Mouritz.
Coward, R. (1989) *The Whole Truth: The Myth of Alternative Health*. London: Faber and Faber.
Crossley, N. (1994) *The Politics of Subjectivity: Between Foucault and Merleau-Ponty*. Aldershot: Avebury.
Crossley, N. (1996) Body-subject/body-power: agency, inscription and control in Foucault and Merleau-Ponty, *Body and Society*, 2, 2, 99–116.
Fischer, J.M. (2008) Letters: BMA members requested study of Alexander Technique in 1937, *British Medical Journal*, 337, a1502. Available at http://www.bmj.com/cgi/content/extract/337/sep10_1/a1502.
Foucault, M. (1973) *The Birth of the Clinic: An Archaeology of Medical Perception*. London: Tavistock Publications.
Foucault, M. (1985) *The Use of Pleasure: The History of Sexuality Volume 2*. New York: Vintage Books.
Foucault, M. (1986) *The Care of the Self: The History of Sexuality Volume 3*. New York: Vintage Books.
Jahoda, G. (1999) *Images of Savages: Ancient Roots of Modern Prejudice in Western Culture*. London and New York: Routledge.
Little, P., Lewith, G., Webley, F., Evans, M., Beattie, A., Middleton, K., Barnett, J., Ballard, K., Oxford, F., Smith, P., Yardley, L., Hollinghurst, S. and Sharp, D. (2008) Randomised control trial of Alexander Technique lessons, exercise, and massage (ATEAM) for chronic and recurrent back pain, *British Medical Journal*, 337: a884. Available at http://bmj.com/cgi/content/full/337/aug19_2/a884, last accessed 14 January 2010.

Merleau-Ponty, M. (1962) *Phenomenology of Perception*. London: Routledge and Kegan Paul.

Oerton, S. and Phoenix, J. (2001) Sex/Bodywork: discourses and practices, *Sexualities*, 4, 4, 387–412.

Rhodes, L.A., McPhillips-Tangum, C.A., Markham, C. and Klenk, R. (1999) The power of the visible: the meaning of diagnostic tests in chronic back pain, *Social Science and Medicine*, 48, 9, 1189–203.

Saks, M. (1994) The alternatives to medicine. In Gabe, J., Kelleher, D. and Williams, G. (eds) *Challenging Medicine*. London/New York: Routledge.

Searle, G.R. (1976) *Eugenics and Politics in Britain 1900–1914*. Leyden, The Netherlands: Noordhoff International Publishing.

Staring, J. (1996) *The First 43 Years of the Life of F. Matthias Alexander: Volume 1*. Nijmegen, The Netherlands: Jeroen Staring.

Staring, J. (1997) *The First 43 Years of the Life of F. Matthias Alexander: Volume 2*. Nijmegen, The Netherlands: Jeroen Staring.

Sharma, U. (1992) *Complementary Medicine Today: Practitioners and Patients*. London and New York: Routledge.

Shilling, C. (2004) *The Body in Culture, Technology and Society*. London: Sage Publications.

Shusterman, R. (2004) The silent, limping body of philosophy. In Carman, T. and Hansen, M.B.N. (eds.) *The Cambridge Companion to Merleau-Ponty*. Cambridge: Cambridge University Press.

Shusterman, R. (2008) *Body Consciousness: A Philosophy of Mindfulness and Somaesthetics*. Cambridge: Cambridge University Press.

Society of Teachers of the Alexander Technique (STAT) (2007) The Definitive Guide to the Alexander Technique provided by STAT – the Society of Teachers of the Alexander Technique. Available at http://www.stat.org.uk/pages/stat.htm, last accessed 18 August 2009.

Tait, R.C. and Chinball, J.T. (1997) Physician judgements of chronic pain patients, *Social Science and Medicine*, 45, 8, 1199–205.

Tarr, J. (2008) Habit and conscious control: ethnography and embodiment in the Alexander Technique, *Ethnography*, 9, 4, 477–97.

Twigg, J. (2000) Carework as a form of bodywork, *Ageing and Society*, 20, 4, 389–411.

Twigg, J. (2004) The spatial ordering of care: public and private in bathing support at home, *Sociology of Health and Illness*, 21, 4, 381–400.

Wiber, M. (1998) *Erect Men/Undulating Women: The Visual Imagery of Gender, 'Race' and Progress in Reconstructive Illustrations of Human Evolution*. Waterloo, ON: Wilfrid Laurier University Press.

Wolkowitz, C. (2002) The social relations of body work, *Work, Employment and Society*, 16, 3, 497–510.

7

Treating women's sexual difficulties: the body work of sexual therapy
Thea Cacchioni and Carol Wolkowitz

Introduction

This chapter explores the interactions of medics and other healthcare practitioners with women's bodies by looking at intervention in the area of women's sexual problems or 'Female Sexual Dysfunction' (FSD), the current medical term for women's difficulties with sexual desire, arousal, orgasm, and pain. While the pharmaceutical industry continues to search for the elusive 'pink Viagra' as a way of 'treating FSD', women seeking advice for sexual problems may be drawn into complex procedures involving close scrutiny, measurement and touch of the genital area by the practitioner. Treatment may also involve instructing the woman patient in genital self-touch. Yet while there is an increasing acceptance of the notion that 'to get to its desired form the body must be touched not only by ourselves but also by others' (Van Dongen and Elema 2001: 153), as yet there is no sociological literature that considers touch in the context of treatment for sexual difficulties.

This chapter looks in detail at sexual therapy for women involving 'body work', *i.e.* work on people's bodies involving touch (Twigg 2000, 2006, Wolkowitz 2002, 2006), as a way of illuminating the power relations between health practitioners and patients and clients. Feminist critics of the medicalisation of sex, along with some commentators on body work in the beauty and weight-loss industries, have tended to see medical practitioners and beauty industry workers as mediators in disciplinary regimes governing women's bodies (Fishman and Mamo 2001, Bartky 1990, Throsby 2004). Other commentators suggest that the power relations of body work are more diverse, being shaped by the relative status of the practitioner or worker and the patient or client (*e.g.* Wolkowitz 2002, Gimlin 2002, Chambliss 1996, Black 2004). However, the salience of touch in these relationships has been highlighted mainly in the study of nursing and care work (*e.g.* Lawler 1997, Twigg 2001).

Treatment for women's sexual difficulties is a particularly interesting example of body work practices, and the expert knowledges they draw on, because the appropriateness of *bodily* intervention in treating women's perceived sexual problems is hotly debated by sexologists, certainly much more so than in most other areas of healthcare. Feminist researchers working in the health and social sciences argue that the concentration on the physiology of sex ignores the socio-political roots of women's sexual dissatisfactions (Kaschak and Tiefer 2001, Cacchioni 2007b, Tiefer 2008). However, this critique focuses on the biochemical solutions touted by the pharmaceutical companies, and has not really considered other

Body Work in Health and Social Care, First Edition. Edited by Julia Twigg, Carol Wolkowitz, Rachel Lara Cohen and Sarah Nettleton.
Chapters © 2011 The Authors. Book compilation © 2011 Foundation for the Sociology of Health & Illness / Blackwell Publishing Ltd. Published 2011 by Blackwell Publishing Ltd.

ways in which practitioners may address the patient's body nor how these techniques might challenge current assumptions about the relation between physiological, psychological and socio-political aspects of sexual difficulties and their treatment.

Treatment for women's sexual difficulties is also distinctive in so far as practitioners may undertake body work of a particularly intimate kind. Up until now it has usually been found that medical practitioners who have to touch women's genitals seek to bypass rather than to engage with the cultural meanings of the vagina, which range from sexual to sacred to abject (Kapsalis 1997). A sizeable literature considers the ways in which practitioners establish touch with women's vaginas during pelvic examinations (although not sexual therapy) (Emerson 1970a, 1970b, Henslin and Biggs 1971, Heath 1986, Kapsalis 1997, Meerabeau 1999, Van Dongen and Elema 2001, Bolton 2005, Stewart 2005, Brown 2011 in this volume). This literature suggests that carefully planned, routinised procedures for 'the management of embarrassment and sexuality in healthcare' (Meerabeau 1999: 1510) seek to evade or dismiss 'general community meanings' about the vagina (Emerson 1970a). Genital touch is often managed through a visual ethic involving techniques such as gaze avoidance and draping.

This chapter concentrates on the treatment of women patients who suffer from sexual pain disorders, which makes intimate touch particularly difficult. Analysing their treatment and their response to it makes it possible to explore the complex, contradictory meanings of genital touch in the case of sexual therapy. Following an explanation of methodology, the first section sets the context by outlining the competing ways in which sexologists and others claiming expertise on female sexuality envision sexuality as an embodied capacity. The second section examines the practices of intimate touch undertaken by therapists, the dilemmas they face, and their reception by their patients or clients. We conclude by considering the goals and methods of these sexual therapies, the challenges that practitioners face, and the implications of all of the above for women, their bodies, and their capacity for sexual enjoyment.

Methodology

This chapter is based on data produced in the first empirical study to date exploring women's experiences of seeking and receiving treatment for perceived sexual difficulties, and practitioners' experiences of conducting treatments (Cacchioni 2007a, 2007b). Most of the fieldwork was undertaken in Vancouver, Canada in 2004, with follow-up research conducted in April 2009. Semi-structured, in-depth interviews were conducted with 31 ethnically diverse women, of whom 28 identify as heterosexual. After obtaining approval from the local university hospital review board, informants were recruited through local community-based advertisements and the co-operation of a hospital-based sexual medicine unit specialising in 'sexual dysfunction'. Interviews lasted 45 minutes to two hours and took place at a time and place of participants' convenience. These women identified as having a range of often overlapping sexual difficulties of desire, arousal, orgasm, and pain, and sought the services of GPs, sexual medicine physicians, pelvic physiotherapists, homeopaths, naturopaths, energy healers, psychiatrists, psychologists, counsellors, sex therapists, and self-help sources. The majority of participants who accessed these services described themselves as 'middle class'.

Because we are defining 'body work' as work in which touching the body is a central component, as in this book as a whole, this chapter draws only on the interviews with women who had received help from healthcare practitioners involving direct touch, chiefly

11 women who attended sexual medicine appointments and 7 women who attended pelvic physiotherapy sessions. Sixteen of this group of 18 struggled with some form of sexual pain, described in greater detail below.

Considering that much of the medical and pharmaceutical research for women experiencing sexual difficulties concentrates on issues affecting postmenopausal women (Berman and Berman 2001), the women in the sample are relatively young. The women who accessed therapies involving touch ranged in age from 24 to 62, with an average of 36, and the women in the study as a whole, who ranged in age from 21 to 62, were even younger, with an average age of 33. While we do not know the reasons for the relative youth of the sample, it may reflect a greater willingness of younger women to respond to requests to participate in a study of this kind.

In-depth interviews were also undertaken with four practitioners who had treated several women in the study, including one sex therapist, two pelvic physiotherapists, and one sexual medicine specialist from the hospital sexual medicine unit mentioned above. All were white women in their late forties. (We have not included information from the interview with the sex therapist, as her practice did not involve direct touch.) The other four physicians employed at the sexual medicine unit did not make themselves available for a one-to-one interview, but they did allow participant observation of six sexual medicine 'rounds' sessions over one year, where doctors discussed their cases and appropriate treatments, developed protocols and had informal discussions.

In addition, observations of pelvic physiotherapy were undertaken. One of the pelvic physiotherapists asked her clients if they would allow a sociologist to observe sessions. The four women whose treatment was observed were all white women in their 20s or 30s, with occupations ranging from secretary to university professor. The physiotherapist explained to them that the sociologist would not reveal their identities and that they could ask her to leave at any time. Understanding the vulnerability women may feel during intimate body work, the researcher sat behind the client's shoulders during examinations and other procedures involving nudity, and recorded her observations after, rather than during, each session. All interview and fieldwork data were transcribed and manually coded by theme with names and identity-revealing information changed.

Debating the importance of the physical body in women's sexual difficulties

The context of treatment for women's sexual difficulties is acrimonious debate over the direction sexology is taking and how this affects women's interests. So far the rights and wrongs of sexologists' understandings of both male and female sexuality have been explored by social scientists mainly in relation to the ways that sexuality is conceptualised and the implications for treatment (*e.g.* Fishman and Mamo 2001, Marshall 2002, Loe 2004, Irvine 1995).

Since the release of Viagra for men's 'erectile dysfunction' (ED) in 1999, there has been increasing research into the physiology of FSD that highlights the place of the body – and in particular vascular, hormonal, and neurological processes – in female sexual response. This includes the search for biochemical solutions to women's sexual difficulties. For instance, at a 2000 conference subtitled 'Desire, Arousal, and Testosterone', founding member of the Boston-based Institute for Sexual Medicine, Dr. Irwin Goldstein, told the audience that he regularly recommends DHEA, an over-the-counter supplement linked to testosterone production, to his women patients. He reported, 'All I can tell you is what I tell my patients – it's like gas in a car. You can't drive unless you have gas. Testosterone is the gas' (Loe 2004: 150).

On the other side, feminist researchers working in the health and social sciences are challenging the concept of FSD as a blanket term that reproduces rather than challenges the social construction of heterosexual sexual norms. Following in the footsteps of earlier feminist critics (*e.g.* Coveney 1984), critics of current sexual science view the importance placed on 'orgasm as endpoint' as at least in part culturally constructed (Jackson and Scott 2001) and often question 'universal claims about normal sexual function' all together (Tiefer 2001).

Leonore Tiefer, who leads 'The Working Group for a New View of Women's Sexual Problems', argues that the current framework for treating women's sexual dissatisfactions is reductionist and androcentric. As she says, 'a framework that reduces sexual problems to disorders of physiological function, comparable to breathing or digestive disorders' (Kaschak and Tiefer 2001: 3) – or indeed, as seen above, to automobile engines – perpetuates 'serious distortions' in the study of female sexuality. Moreover, an apparently 'gender neutral' model, as in much current sexology, may disguise gender inequality and obscure differences in male and female sexual responses.

The 'New View' stresses that it recognises the existence of 'medical conditions', for instance sexual pain or lack of physical response, mainly if such problems occur 'despite [the existence of] a supportive and safe interpersonal situation' (Kaschak and Tiefer 2001: 6). However, Tiefer acknowledges that sexual-pain conditions, in particular, have tended to fall off its agenda (Tiefer 2005). Understandably because the 'New View' commentators have prioritised the need to challenge the narrow focus on the physiology of women's sexual problems in the medical literature, less attention has been paid to what should be done about the bodily dimension of sexual dissatisfactions.

Touching women's bodies

While medical and other scholarly debates regarding female sexual problems rage, women who see themselves as having sexual problems continue to seek 'expert' advice, without necessarily knowing very much about these differences of opinion. A handful of cities in the US boast highly specialised private clinics designed specifically to treat 'FSD', for example, the 'Wellness Centers' owned and operated by Jennifer Berman, who studied at the Boston Institute for Sex Research, and her sister (Berman Sexual Health 2009). At these clinics, women may be assessed using a range of equipment designed to assess 'vaginal elasticity', 'clitoral sensation', and 'pelvic blood flow', as well as probes described by manufacturers as 'intra-vaginal vibratory insertion units'.

In Vancouver, however, the only practitioners who deal directly with women's bodies in treatments for their perceived sexual difficulties are sexual medicine specialists, working within the public healthcare system, and pelvic physiotherapists, working in private practice. These practitioners do not use the highly technological devices listed above to assess and measure women's bodies. For the most part, they use direct touch, although pelvic physiotherapists also use a device called a 'biofeedback machine', described below. It is typically women's sexual pain problems that are treated with methods that involve touch (although touch may also be involved in the diagnosis of other difficulties).

Whether these methods are widely available elsewhere is difficult to estimate. The extent of provision is not dealt with in the medical literature evaluating the rehabilitation of the pelvic floor in treatment of chronic pelvic pain leading to sexual pain (Rosenbaum 2007) nor in the few existing studies of women's accounts of living with chronic pelvic pain (Kaler 2006, Ayling and Ussher 2008), which do not deal with women's experiences of treatment.

The Vancouver study indicated that women experiencing sexual pain actively sought expert advice. Of the eleven participants who obtained access to the sexual medicine unit of the hospital, nine had issues with sexual pain, one had problems with orgasm and one with arousal. These women waited an average of six months to see a specialist. The seven participants who obtained pelvic physiotherapy, all of whom had sexual pain issues, waited an average of three months. The services of the sexual medicine unit are covered by Canada's universal health insurance scheme, but since 2001 many physiotherapy services have been excluded. Hence, women without private health insurance must pay up to $175 (CDN) for each pelvic physiotherapy session.

The medical approach to touching women's bodies
Sexual medicine is a medical subfield comprising physicians who were originally trained as general practitioners, gynaecologists, or psychiatrists. Still striving for legitimacy, sexual medicine specialists face a difficult career path. Although the Vancouver-based sexual medicine unit was established in the 1970s, it did not offer a paid residency program in sexual medicine until the 1990s. The sexual medicine specialist interviewed said that she had struggled to obtain training and that the unit still has to fight for support. She adds that 'Sex is often swept under the carpet' in the wider medical profession, and that sexual medicine is particularly vulnerable to funding cuts. Of the politics of healthcare funding she remarks, 'Now that everyone is fighting for their existence, we've been advised to be a bit more public because [. . .] we could be chopped, and who will make a noise for us?'

The three women physicians in the sexual medicine unit, who originally trained as GPs or gynaecologists, deal with physical complaints related to sexual functioning and two male physicians originally trained as psychiatrists address what they classify as purely psychological issues. Therefore, only the women doctors in this unit deal directly with women's bodies. The conditions they treat offer insight into the multitude of physiological issues that their patients present, including sexual difficulties related to Parkinson's disease, Multiple Sclerosis, spinal cord injuries, vaginal thinning due to menopause and 'iatrogenic conditions' caused by anti-depressants, chemotherapy, and pelvic surgery. In particular, they specialise in treating sexual pain conditions. Many of their patients with sexual pain problems suffer from chronic pelvic pain conditions such as 'vestibulodynia', formerly called vulvar vestibulitis, (Murina *et al.* 2008) which the doctors claim was caused by skin irritations, childbirth-related injuries, or genetic factors.

Despite their focus on physiological issues affecting sexual enjoyment, the sexual medicine physicians claimed to follow a 'biopsychosocial' model for understanding women's sexual problems. Psychosocial issues such as patients' experiences of sexual violence, low self- esteem, poor body image, and the stress of women's double shift were acknowledged during hospital rounds presentations and discussions. However, it was also clear that the physicians saw their role as restoring physiological 'sexual functioning', without challenging this psychosocial context. For instance, they often prescribed drugs, such as testosterone pills and creams, and also did research on the efficacy of various medications. What were explicitly classified as psychological issues were usually dealt with separately, being allocated to the in-house psychiatrists, who would typically see patients for a few sessions and then refer them to counsellors or therapists outside the sexual medicine unit.

Mirroring early findings by Emerson (1970a, 1970b), discussions in sexual medicine rounds meetings revealed a clear contradiction between the notion that the vagina was a body part like any other and the idea that this body part must be approached with extreme care. Doctors discussed examining the vagina, as they would any other body part, for signs of measurable conditions, using terms such as 'variable redness', 'vaginal tears', pain upon 'opening', and 'stretching' or 'allodynia', and 'painful response to non-painful touch'. They talked about arousal, lubrication, and orgasm in the same way they would discuss other bodily functions. At the same time, they realised that they must overcome the potential for legal challenges, embarrassment, physical discomfort, and other issues arising from body work focused on the vagina. Therefore, during hospital rounds meetings, the specialists, including the psychiatrists, developed protocols for establishing boundaries while touching women intimately. These included draping techniques, using verbal instruction to alert women to what they would be doing before doing it, and offering women the option of having a chaperone. They also discussed what to do if 'a patient becomes involuntarily aroused during the clinical process'. One of the doctors suggested 'Move away, stop, and have a face-to-face discussion about it'.

The sexual medicine specialists also struggled to overcome the challenge of touching women's vaginas in cases where touch may cause physical pain or extreme anxiety. This is because women's chronic pelvic pain is typically accompanied by 'vaginismus', a 'fear and tightening response to vaginal penetration' (Leiblum 2000). In most cases, vaginismus is part and parcel of an existing pelvic pain condition and this is sometimes treated with pain medication. Less often women have the symptoms of vaginismus without a pre-existing painful condition. In these cases, they were seen as having an 'irrational phobia' of penetration, for some women by a penis only, but for others by a tampon or any other object. Whether the vaginismus was caused by a fear reaction due to the experience of ongoing pelvic pain, as it was for thirteen participants, or had less obvious origins, as it was for three participants, the medics saw it as a physical manifestation of a 'psychological issue', but one that could be addressed by hands-on body work. In all these cases, treatment for vaginismus is seen as necessarily requiring direct touch of the body and, due to the nature of the symptoms, touch must be negotiated with extreme care. Hence, in practice, the treatment of vaginismus, and occasionally other complaints, transcends the usual division between physical and psychological sexual problems.

The sexual medicine specialists used a slow, gradual, approach to treating vaginismus, emphasising the patient's active participation in clinical procedures and sexual activities. The specialists interviewed said that they had developed some of these 'common sense' procedures themselves, drawing on their experience 'as women'. These procedures were developed initially as a way of making a pelvic examination possible, but, according to one specialist, she soon realised the therapeutic benefits of the approach she had adopted. In order to ease the patients into the experience of being touched, they begin the process with pre-clinical exam 'homework'. As the specialist interviewed explains, 'We'll wait until she's done a little bit more self-touch before we actually attempt to see what's actually going on in the vagina'. She may also prescribe pre-exam exercises including 'kegel exercises, relaxation techniques, and bearing down techniques' which enhance women's capacity to control their own vaginas.[1] The initial exam itself is designed with 'therapeutic' as well as diagnostic intentions. 'It's not conducted like a routine such as a Pap smear. It's done much more slowly', with the woman actively participating in the process. While the patient sits up holding a mirror, the physician explains the functions of various parts of the vagina and then leads her through variations on a kegel exercise. The interviewed physician explains the rationale for this approach:

She's feeling like, you know, 'I'm not just having this done to me'. You know it's not enough to tell her that she can tell me when to stop anytime. It's a lot easier if she's right there and to have her help as much as possible. Her spreading the labia is much better, for one, it's much easier, you've still got two hands left! And number two, you know, that's permission for you to go ahead. I mean, there's nothing clearer than saying to her, 'Okay take a look'. It means she's doing. She's helping. And they are much rougher on themselves than I am.

Once the patient is comfortable with being touched by the doctor and/or herself, the doctor asks the patient to 'tighten and withdraw', doing a range of kegel and reverse kegel exercises so that women can see that 'Oh my goodness, I can control this'. The patient is then asked to insert her own finger into her vulva or to insert the doctor's finger, whichever she is more comfortable with. Even so, 'Some of them get quite faint if they have never been looked at or touched before, even if you're going very gently and very slowly, in tiny steps. She may become very dizzy so you want to get her down [on a couch] quickly'.

Once the patient with vaginismus is seen as ready to attempt penetration, she is prescribed vaginal dilators, invented by Masters and Johnson, or vaginal accommodators as they are sometimes called. These tapered, wax candle-like objects are graduated in diameter. Women are encouraged to spend time with these devices at home, graduating to a full-size, penis- shaped dildo, and then to 'the real thing'. When the doctor and patient agree that the patient is ready to accept a penis into her vagina, if that is her goal, the physician gives her careful instructions on how to ease into this process. In her own words, she tells her vaginisums patients, 'See if one day you can't just sit on him a little bit. Look, if you're sitting on him, you're totally in control. Even sit on him a little bit. Or a bit more. Then come right off again.' As she explains, 'It's important that they feel in control and that rather than thinking she's going to be entered, pierced, penetrated by this object that's going to be painful, that actually she's going to learn how to control her vagina and the opening of her vagina'. The doctor suggests that the key is for the woman to understand that penetration is an active, not a passive, process. She wants her patient to see 'that she can actually choose to kind of envelop something, surround something, [. . .] actively. She can choose to tighten up and withdraw, she can choose not to tighten up and withdraw'.

The pelvic physiotherapy approach to touching women's bodies
Pelvic physiotherapy, also referred to as urogynaecological physiotherapy, is a sub-discipline of physiotherapy. With its close focus on sex and the body, like sexual medicine and other body work involving the vagina, it is also a difficult career path to pursue. Both pelvic physiotherapists sought training in Britain, Australia, or the US, where pelvic physiotherapy is better established, and at the time of writing there is still no formal institutional training for such a career in Canada. One physio explained that it is not a popular specialism with physiotherapy students, because students have to practise doing pelvic examinations and other body work procedures on each other.

The pelvic physiotherapists interviewed for this study were adamant that their clients' difficulties with penetration stemmed primarily from physical problems causing vaginal pain. They listed these issues as childbirth-related injuries, spinal cord injuries, postoperative scarring of the vaginal tissues, endometriosis, skin sensitivities, gastrointestinal problems, bowel problems, or urinary incontinence. The basic theory of pelvic physiotherapy is that any of these physiological problems can lead to an involuntary tightening of the pelvic floor, making penetrative sex painful. For the most part, the practitioners applied the laws of muscle function and pain pathophysiology research conducted on other body parts to the vagina, theorising that attempted painful intercourse sets off a neurological pain alarm system, making pain even worse. They do not entirely ignore psychological issues influencing women's sexual problems, but their focus is on the body, seeing psychological stress as a consequence of bodily discomfort or pain during sex. They view their treatments as complementing whatever drug therapies the client has been prescribed for sexual pain by their doctors.

Treatment by pelvic physiotherapists encourages women to become aware of their pain triggers (diet, movement, times during a menstrual cycle, sexual activity); to understand exactly where they feel pain; to learn how to strengthen the pelvic floor muscle; to learn how to relax the pelvic floor muscles; finally, to be able to recognise when these muscles are tense or relaxed. They acknowledge that all of the above are tricky, since women in general 'aren't aware of that part of their anatomy' and rarely discuss how it should feel 'normally'. For example, some women with pelvic pain might think that sexual intercourse, or simply inserting a tampon, is supposed to be somewhat painful. Like the sexual medicine physicians, the pelvic physiotherapists are also aware that touching the vagina can be legally contentious if done inappropriately. One admitted, 'I was very, very concerned in the beginning about anybody saying there was misconduct or anything', but 'I've been surprised' that such issues 'have not been a problem at all'.

Three processes involve direct touch of the body in pelvic physiotherapy: examination, biofeedback, and pelvic massage. Acknowledging that 'It's not easy to sit here with your clothes off for half an hour with someone poking around your vagina', the pelvic physiotherapists take extreme care when touching this body part. Beginning with the examination process, the physiotherapist observed in this study attempts to 'make my clients feel comfortable' and to 'set clear boundaries'. After taking a detailed history, she leaves the room, asking them to undress. She tells them, 'Here's the sheet, when you're done undressing, lie down on your back with your head on the pillow and here's a sheet you can cover yourself with'. She explains, 'A lot of people want to scoot down' but 'physios examine differently than physicians'. When she returns, she lets the client lie still with the sheet fully covering her body as a means of relaxation. She begins the exam by exposing the woman's belly and watching her breathe. Only then will she expose the vagina below the sheet, describing what she is doing as she goes along. She comments, 'It's gradual; it's only as needed.

Before she begins touching anywhere in the pelvic region, the physiotherapist emphasises, 'If, at any time you want me to stop, just let me know. If you're uncomfortable, so am I'. She then dons a glove and begins the internal examination, describing every step of the way where she is touching and what she is doing. To test muscle function, she asks clients to do a kegel while the practitioner inserts a finger into the vulva and/or the anus. If they are unable to master this lying down, she asks them to stand up, 'pigeon-toed, make sure your draping covers your bum'. She then inserts her finger into their vulva and/or anus and asks them to contract and release. In cases where patients with vulvar pain are extremely anxious, she may use Xlocaine, a numbing gel to de-sensitise them. Though no crying was witnessed during observation, the physiotherapist said that it often occurs during this procedure. In this case she would stop and give the client a break or the option of finishing for the day. However, most women ask to continue.

The next step is biofeedback, a method used in all physiotherapy specialisms to raise people's awareness of, and ability to relax, an injured body part. It involves connecting the targeted body part to a computer using a sensory device, allowing the subject to visualise movements in that body part. Through a simple line graph, the computer screen displays the tensing and relaxation of this body part, which helps the client understand what 'tensed' or 'relaxed' feels like in an area where tension has become so normalised for her that she does not recognise it. In pelvic physiotherapy, the vagina is connected to the biofeedback machine either by electrodes placed on the thigh and anus or with a sensory device inserted into the vulva. Movements are guided by specific exercises such as kegel and reverse kegel exercises designed to tense and relax the pelvic floor muscles. The biofeedback readout displays a flat line when muscles are relaxed, sharp peaks and valleys when they are not. In more advanced sessions with women who were nearing the end of their treatment, the physiotherapist asks them to create different kinds of lines on the screen by tensing or relaxing their pelvic floor muscles in different ways. For approximately 20 minutes she asks them to do a series of 'ramps', 'spikes', 'gentle releases', and 'releases'.

Another pelvic physiotherapy method is pelvic massage, though there is debate over its effectiveness. One of the physiotherapists used this method, massaging the pelvic floor muscles internally and externally in order to 'loosen' the area and soften and stretch the tissue. Pelvic massage also incorporates 'trigger point work', touching women's vaginas, in her words, 'below the pain threshold'. In her opinion, this eased the process of penile-vaginal penetration and desensitised painful areas. As she explains, 'You're working with the muscles, you're making sure that they're lengthened, that they're not in spasm, they are able to relax, that they can get stronger. But you're also dealing with very reactive muscles so that when you touch them, they can go like this [making a fist]'.

Women's responses to treatments involving touch
How did the participants in this study who identify as having sexual difficulties evaluate the body work sexual therapy they have received? Their perceptions of sexual touch seems to depend vitally on the ability of the practitioner to (1) take physiological complaints seriously; (2) develop slow, gradual, and careful methods for touching the body; and (3) create methods in which the patient could actively participate in the process as active spectators.

Participants in this study liked the 'hands-on' attention they received during treatment in sexual medicine and pelvic physiotherapy, because to them this meant their bodily complaints were being taken seriously by an 'expert'. The women in this study who were eventually referred to the sexual medicine unit or to a pelvic physiotherapist were thrilled with the careful attention their bodies were given. The majority of them claimed to have previously encountered general practitioners or non-sexual medicine gynaecologists who either 'ignored' or 'dismissed' their physical concerns or, in some cases, failed to approach their bodies carefully.

The account provided by Courtney, a student aged 25 who identified as having vaginismus illustrates this point. Like many women with an intense fear of penetration, Courtney was referred to a non-sexual medicine gynaecologist who failed miserably at the task of approaching her body. He first promised her that 'he just wanted to look and see' but 'he just started poking away [. . .] and eventually tried to put his finger inside'. Courtney 'screamed' because 'it was so horrible and painful'. The gynaecologist responded to her lack of compliance by saying, 'You know, if you can't let me do this then I can't help you'. He advised her to try using 'birthday candles' or 'a carrot' to retrain her body. Courtney contrasts this to the careful approach taken to touching her body when she was treated at the sexual medicine unit of the hospital. Her sexual medicine specialist at the unit 'made it really clear that I didn't *have* to do anything. We'll do it at your own pace'. Ironically, when her sexual medicine physician prescribed vaginal dilators, she saw this in positive terms, despite the fact that dilators are actually not very different from wax candles in size or shape.

Just as a visual ethic of avoidance characterises traditional pelvic exams (Henslin and Biggs 1971, Heath 1986), a visual ethic of looking is part and parcel of the development of empowering body work techniques. While women have been encouraged to look at their vaginas as a way of reappropriating the male medical gaze since the early days of the women's health movement (Davis 2007), 'self-spectatorship is virtually unaccounted for in the traditional gynecological theatre' (Kapsalis 1997: 166). However, it seems that practitioners specialising in treating women's sexual problems have caught on to the power of active spectatorship to enhance women's capacity for sexual enjoyment. Participants valued the use of visual methods such as mirrors or biofeedback. This process of 'looking' was seen as increasing their sense of control and awareness of their own bodies. For instance, Lindsay, a 39-year-old woman with sexual arousal problems, referred to her physician in this unit as 'awesome' because 'Rather than the standard "Put your legs up, lay back, throw a towel over your face" approach, I was told, "You can sit right up and take a look with me"'. As Lindsay remarked, 'Just getting patient involvement . . . was really cool' and also 'more comfortable'. Samantha, a 24-year-old woman with orgasm problems, found this visual approach educational, explaining that her physician 'pointed to different spots and parts that are good for stimulation'. Linda, aged 22, similarly noted, 'I used to think I peed out of my clitoris [. . .] So, definitely the mirror was an amazing teaching tool for her to teach me what was going on'. Charlene agreed, reflecting that 'Most women have never even looked down there, so they don't know what they're supposed to be looking at'.

The visual-physical feedback loop displayed on the biofeedback machine screen was also prized. Participants explained how it helped them interpret their bodily sensations. Consider these comments by two women in their twenties who have been diagnosed with vaginismus:

> It was helpful because it was very educational how much your muscles will tense up as a result of painful sex or actual pain [. . .] You could see the activity of the muscles, [what] the tone of your muscles was, so if they were tight, you could see that on the screen and then see when you're relaxing them. And so to have the actual feedback was very helpful [. . .] You could feel your body relaxing and you see it happening and so as a result you're in better control of it.

> It [having the biofeedback] meant that I have much greater awareness of what relaxed feels like. And it doesn't feel like being relaxed. It feels kind of like pushing. And I wasn't aware of that before. It means that I can consciously relax. I think that all of that has to do with building control.

Conclusions

At the time of writing, a 'pink Viagra' has yet to be invented to address women's perceived sexual difficulties. Some sexual therapy practitioners, in this case, sexual medicine specialists and physiotherapists, continue to offer body work services to address women's immediate complaints of sexual pain. The sexual medicine specialists conduct educational pelvic exams and prescribe various body work exercises for the vagina, while the pelvic physiotherapists teach women about their vaginas through biofeedback, and, even more intimately, some administer pelvic massage. Each of these practitioners attends to women's immediate complaints of sexual discomfort or displeasure through forms of body work that encourage women to feel in control during both body work procedures and sexual activities. Their clients and patients may present with a number of physiological complaints, but their treatments have the effect of enhancing women's connections to and control over their vaginas.

These data on a particular form of sexual therapy support the general tenor of the feminist critique of the medicalisation of sex. For instance, there are clearly important ways in which the sexual therapies discussed here reproduce normative heterosexuality. In so far as they are intended to allow women to participate in penetrative intercourse, they do not challenge either the heteronormative framework of what 'real' sex is (Jackson and Scott

2001) or the notion that we must all be sexual (Loe 1999). Nor do they challenge the notion that women and their healthcare practitioners (rather than men) are ultimately responsible for the work involved in managing heterosexual relationships (Cacchioni 2007b). It is also an individualising approach. Whether or not these practitioners recognise the social context of women's sexual problems in similar terms as the feminist 'New View', they see themselves as most effective in using their skills to help women overcome, individually, their sexual difficulties. Just as Haraway (1999) saw the 1970s women's self-help movement as empowering individual middle-class women, rather than seeking to transform the wider politics of healthcare, so it could be argued that these practitioners operate largely within current conventions of healthcare and heterosexuality, rather than promoting a collective challenge to the current state of sexual politics.

Nonetheless, looking in detail at the body work undertaken by these practitioners suggests that it accords with feminist thinking in important ways. The body workers described in this chapter accomplish some of the objectives of 1970s consciousness-raising efforts aimed at encouraging women to 'get in touch with their bodies' (Davis 2007) and parallel the emphasis on women's ability to pleasure themselves seen in the current explosion of feminist sex shops (Loe 1999). It is not simply that sexual therapy body work procedures encourage women to overcome sexual shame, anxiety, and discomfort quite literally by facing their vaginas. It is also that they challenge 'phallocentrism' (Smart 1989) by treating the vagina as an active organ, rather than as a passive receptacle awaiting a male penis with inevitable pleasure. Sexual therapy of the kind discussed here also challenges heterosexual romantic discourse in which the woman naturally 'falls into a man's arms' and accepts him utterly.

The women patients' views also counter critiques of biomedicine insofar as those who were able to access specialist sexual therapy body work procedures described the body work techniques as therapeutic and empowering. For instance, they said that they found the visualisation techniques adopted by the practitioners helped them to connect to their bodies, rather than feeling that the techniques objectified them. This supports other research that has found that imaging techniques are not normally experienced by patients as alienating, especially when the patient is able to see and discuss the images as they are produced (Blaxter 2009). Moreover, the treatments administered by practitioners offering hands-on care were highly prized by women patients and clients for a careful, slow, gradual, approach which encouraged women to be active participants in the overall process. The practitioners' carefully thought-out processes have come a long way from the 'dehumanizing' pelvic exams described by Henslin and Biggs' (1971) classic account. Rather, they may reflect a recent movement to 'humanize' touch in intimate healthcare. As Van Dongen and Elema (2001) note, while individuals are increasingly happy to 'surrender to the touch of others', they also exercise 'reflexive concern about personal control and personal space' (2001: 153).

It would seem, therefore, that commentators perhaps too readily assume that 'biomedical treatment regimes', such as those that focus on 'muscle hypertonicity in the vulva', ignore 'psychological or relational issues' (Ayling and Ussher 2008: 295) or take place in a social vacuum. Treatments that deal with the body are not necessarily limited, in application or effect, to physiological functioning. This suggests the need, whether with respect to sexual difficulties or more generally, to stress the usefulness of seeing different types of work on the body as forms of social interaction, not merely physical interventions, with many possible ramifications.

Close attention to the body work of sexual therapy also brings new perspectives to bear on professional roles. Sexual therapists involved in body work procedures seem to occupy an awkward place within healthcare, perhaps related to the association between dealing with the vagina and 'dirty work', moral and physical (Bolton 2005, Twigg 2006). In addition, both groups of practitioners have evolved therapeutic practices that cross professional divisions. Whereas Wolkowitz (2002) presumed there were big differences in the ways high-ranking doctors and lower-ranked practitioners dealt with patients' bodies, the similarities between the approaches of these medics and physiotherapists are striking. Although both groups must infringe women's bodily privacy, at the same time they work to enhance patients' or clients' sense of control over their bodies; and they help women to navigate the paradox of working towards pleasure despite pain, discomfort, or anxiety. It may be that in this relatively new area of practice, in which knowledge is not yet rigidified, practitioners have been able to evolve their own methods and protocols on the basis of their own experiences as women and as therapists.

A female Viagra equivalent, if even a possibility, cannot possibly replace these hands-on interactions and visual techniques and the value women attach to them. Seemingly, the pharmaceutical approach to treating women's sexual difficulties would leave out key steps in a highly tactile process that involves the therapeutic power of embodied touch and empowered looking. These body work interactions between female practitioner and patient seem to help women with the privilege of access to these resources to understand and accept the ways in which their vaginas look, feel, and function. Embodied understanding and acceptance could be the most potent drug of all when it comes to women's sexual enjoyment.

Note

1   A kegel exercise consists of contracting and relaxing one's own pelvic floor muscles

References

Ayling, K. and Ussher, J.M. (2008) 'If sex hurts am I still a woman?' The subjective experience of vulvodynia, *Archives of Sexual Behavior*, 37, 1, 294–304.
Bartky, S.L. (1990) *Femininity and Domination*. New York: Routledge.
Berman Sexual Health 2009. Accessed at www.bermansexualhealth.com.
Berman, J., Berman, L. and with Bumiller, E. (2001) *For Women Only: a Revolutionary Guide to Reclaiming Your Sex Life*. New York: Henry Holt and Co.
Black, P. (2004) *The Beauty Industry*. London: Routledge.
Blaxter. M. (2009) The case of the vanishing patient: image and experience, *Sociology of Health and Illness*, 3, 5, 762–78.
Bolton, S.C. (2005) Women's work, dirty work: the gynaecology nurse as 'Other', *Gender, Work and Organization*, 12, 2, 169–86.
Cacchioni, T. (2007a) *Female Sexual Dysfunction: the Medicalization of Heterosex in the Post Viagra Age*. Doctoral Dissertation, University of Warwick.
Cacchioni, T. (2007b) Successful heterosexuality and 'the labour of love': a contribution to recent debates on female sexual dysfunction, *Sexualities*, 10, 3, 299–320.
Chambliss, D. (1996) *Beyond Caring*. Chicago: University of Chicago Press.
Coveney, L. (1984) *The Sexuality Papers: Male Sexuality and the Social Control of Women*. London: Hutchinson.
Davis, K. (2007) Reclaiming women's bodies, *The Sociological Review*, 55, 1, 50–64.
Emerson, J. (1970a) Nothing unusual happening. In Shibutani, T. (ed.) *Human Nature and Collective Behaviour*. Englewood Cliffs: Prentice Hall.
Emerson, J. (1970b) Behaviour in private places: sustaining definitions of reality in gynecological examinations. In Dreitzel, H. (ed.) *Recent Sociology*. New York: Macmillan.

Fishman, J.R. and Mamo, L. (2001) What's in a disorder? A cultural analysis of medical and phar-maceutical constructions of male and female sexual dysfunction. In Kaschak, E. and Tiefer, L. (eds) *A New View of Women's Sexual Problems*. Binghamton: The Haworth Press.

Gimlin, D.L. (2002) *Body Work: Beauty and Self-image in American Culture*. Berkeley: University of California Press.

Haraway, D. (1999) The virtual speculum in the new world order. In Clarke, A. and Olesen, V. (eds) *Revisioning Women, Health, and Healing*. New York: Routledge.

Heath, C, (1986) *Body Movement and Speech in Medical Interaction*. Cambridge: Cambridge University Press.

Henslin, J. and Biggs, M. (1971) Dramaturgical desexualisation: the sociology of the vaginal examina-tion. In Henslin, J. (ed.) *Studies in the Sociology of Sex*. New York: Appleton Century Crofts.

Irvine, J. (1995) Regulated passions: the diversion of inhibited sexual desire and sexual addiction. In Terry, J. and Urla, J. (eds) *Deviant Bodies*. Indiana: Indiana University Press.

Jackson, S. and Scott, S. (2001) Embodying orgasm: gendered power relations and sexual pleasure. In Kaschak, E. and Tiefer, L. (eds) *A New View of Women's Sexual Problems*. Binghamton: The Haworth Press.

Kaler, A. (2006) Unreal women: sex, gender, identity and the lived experience of vulvar pain, *Feminist Review*, 82, 1, 50–75.

Kapsalis, T. (1997) *Public Privates: Performing Gynecology from Both Ends of the Speculum*. Durham, N.C. and London: Duke University Press.

Kaschak, E. and Tiefer, L. (eds) (2001) *A New View of Women's Sexual Problems*. Binghamton: The Haworth Press.

Lawler, J. (ed.) (1997) *The Body in Nursing*. South Melbourne: Churchill Livingston.

Leiblum, S. (2000) Vaginismus: a most perplexing problem. In Leiblum, S. and Rosen, R. (eds) *Principles and Practices of Sex Therapy*. New York: Guilford Press.

Lin, Y.L. and Taylor, A.G. (1998) Effects of therapeutic touch in reducing pain and anxiety in an elderly population, *Integrative Medicine*, 1, 4, 155–62.

Loe, M. (1999) Feminism for sale: case study of a pro-sex feminist business, *Gender and Society*, 13, 6, 705–32.

Loe, M. (2004) *The Rise of Viagra: How the Little Blue Pill Changed Sex In America*. New York: New York University Press.

Marshall, B. (2002) 'Hard science': gendered constructions of sexual dysfunction in the 'Viagra Age,' *Sexualities*, 5, 2, 131–58.

Meerabeau, L. (1999) The management of embarrassment and sexuality in healthcare, *The Journal of Advanced Nursing*, 29, 6, 1507–13.

Murina, F., Bernorio, R. and Palmiotto, R. (2008) Amielle vaginal trainers as adjuvant in the treat-ment of vestibulodynia: an observational multicentric study, *The Medscape Journal of Medicine*, 10, 1, 23.

Nicolson, P. (1993) Deconstructing sexology: the pathologization of female sexuality, *Journal of Reproductive and Infant Psychology*, 11, 4, 191–201.

Rosenbaum, T.Y. (2007) Pelvic floor involvement in male and female sexual dysfunction and the role of pelvic floor rehabilitation in treatment: a Literature Review, *Journal of Sexual Medicine*, 4, 4–13.

Smart, C. (1989) *Feminism and the Power of Law*. London: Routledge.

Stewart, M. (2005) 'I'm going to wash you down': sanitizing the vaginal examination, *Journal of Advanced Nursing*, 51, 6, 587–94.

The Working Group for a New View of Women's Sexual Problems (2001) A New View of Women's Sexual Problems. In Kaschak, E. and Tiefer, L. (eds) *A New View of Women's Sexual Problems*. Binghamton: The Haworth Press.

Throsby, K. (2004) *When IVF Fails*. Basingstoke: Palgrave Macmillan.

Tiefer, L. (2001). Arriving at a 'New View' of women's sexual problems: background, theory, and activism. In Kaschak, E. and Tiefer, L. (eds) *A New View of Women's Sexual Problems*. Binghamton: The Haworth Press.

Tiefer, L. (2005) Dyspareunia is the only valid sexual dysfunction, *Archives of Sexual Behavior*, 34, 49–51.

Tiefer, L. (2008). *Sex is Not a Natural Act and Other Essays*. 2nd Edition. Boulder: Westview Press.

Twigg, J. (2000) Carework as a form of bodywork, *Ageing and Society*, 20, 389–411.

Twigg, J. (2001) *Bathing – the Body and Community Care*. London: Routledge.

Twigg, J. (2006) *The Body in Health and Social Care*. Basingstoke: Palgrave Macmillan.

Van Dongen, E. and Elema, R. (2001) The art of touching: the culture of 'body work' in nursing, *Anthropology and Medicine*, 8, 2/3, 149–62.

Wolkowitz, C. (2002).The social relations of body work, *Work, Employment and Society*, 16, 3, 497–510.

Wolkowitz, C. (2006) *Bodies at Work*. London: Sage.

...s speak louder than words: the embodiment of trust by healthcare professionals in gynae-oncology

Patrick R. Brown, Andy Alaszewski, Trish Swift and Andy Nordin

Introduction

The provision of 'holistic' care by health professionals has been seen as increasingly signifi-cant for quality outcomes. This broadening of focus is driven partly by consumerist tenden-cies within healthcare policy and the resulting import attached to the 'patient- experience', but at a more instrumental level through a growing awareness (following Cohen and Lazarus 1973 amongst others) of the links between minimising anxiety/stress and post-intervention outcomes. The emergence of trust as a key concept for both policy-makers (*e.g.* Department of Health 2007) and those carrying out healthcare research (Brownlie *et al.* 2008) can be partly understood in these terms. For trust has been conceptualised as facilitating positive dispositions towards healthcare providers at both the micro- and macro-levels (Taylor-Gooby 2008) as well as an ' "emotional inoculation" against anxiety' (Elliott 2004: 73).

In spite of the affective aspects of trust and the function of medicine in tending to the problematic body, discussions of the concept (not least in relation to healthcare) have remained notably 'disembodied'. Perhaps this is unsurprising, given conceptions of trust in terms of the truster's beliefs about the *competence* and *care* of the expert professional (*e.g.* Poortinga and Pidgeon 2003, Calnan and Rowe 2008) and prevailing understandings of these latter attributes. Professional competence has increasingly come to be seen as the effective application of abstract, encoded knowledge rather than a tacit, tactile craft (Sennett 2008, Nettleton *et al.* 2008). Moreover motivations (benevolent/caring or otherwise) are typically understood as abstract agendas (Williams 2007), for example in 'putting the patient first', and the truth or validity claims around these (Habermas 1987: 280). So whilst recent research into trust and healthcare emphasises the over-arching importance of patient/professional interactions for trust (Harrison and Smith 2004, Brown 2008, 2009), the purpose of this chapter is to underline the innately embodied nature of such communication. In this way, trust is based on far more than mere speech acts but rather invokes a much more physical and multi-sensory 'presentation of self' (Goffman 1959).

This consideration of trust has important implications for body work and its impact on the service-user – particularly how, in spanning different moments in time, trust moreover

Body Work in Health and Social Care, First Edition. Edited by Julia Twigg, Carol Wolkowitz, Rachel Lara Cohen and Sarah Nettleton.
Chapters © 2011 The Authors. Book compilation © 2011 Foundation for the Sociology of Health & Illness / Blackwell Publishing Ltd. Published 2011 by Blackwell Publishing Ltd.

links seemingly distinct facets of body work. Of central concern are the modes by which body work as 'the management of embodied emotional experience and display' (Gimlin 2007: 353), in the more immediate context, characterises perceptions of body work as 'paid labour carried out on the bodies of others' (2007: 353) in the future. The unique setting of gynae-oncology – for those receiving either treatment or preventative assessment/interventions – makes for a pertinent case study. The way this specialism involves the threat posed by the cancerous tumour to (feminine) personhood (Shilling 2008: 124) on the one hand, and the liminality between the internal and external body (Grosz 1994: 79) on the other, heightens the salience of the 'latent intentionality' (Merleau-Ponty 1968: 213) of the (typically male) clinician, as inferred through embodied interactions with the female patient. While Merleau-Ponty does not emphasise the significance of gender for this *reading* of intentions, the gendered nature of inter-personal interactions and the way these relate to gendered expectations of the broader medical role ('how a doctor ought to appear/act') is highly salient here[1].

The following section will present a more in-depth theoretical consideration of this embodied experience of gynaecological cancer and its ramifications for a body work which is able to win trust. From this conceptual basis (and following a brief account of the research approach and method) three key aspects of body work, as it bears upon trust, will be considered in the light of data from interviews with gynae-oncology patients. First, linkages between the 'communicative body' (physical presentation-of-self as a mode of conveying information) of the present and the body work of the future, and even the past, will be explored – in the light of the theoretical exposition and through the qualitative data.

The second section underlines the role of communication for trust and its verbal and non-verbal nature. Building on this holistic/embodied conception of trust, patients' accounts suggested the absence of a neat dualism between the verbal and non-verbal. Instead a complex summation of signs combined to form an approximation of an 'ideal-type' (Schutz 1972) of trustworthy professional, as made possible through common under-standings (Hindmarsh and Heath 2000). Or rather in some cases, a number of facets, such as posture, eye contact and other physical presentations combined with verbal signs to undermine trust within these intimate clinical situations/examinations. Thirdly, it became apparent that for a number of patients it was specific actions/gestures which were most vital in winning or undermining trust. So whilst verbal signs were still a feature and connected to clarifying the agendas along which trust was worked out, the actions (more so than words) were seemingly decisive in substantiating the likely competence and care of the clinician.

Connecting body work to the patient experience: a multi-dimensional and multi-temporal phenomenon

Relating trust to a 'sociology of the body' is far from novel. Indeed, one of the pre-eminent thinkers behind the invigoration of the body as a key locus of analysis (O'Neill 1972) posits the attitudes of the lay person, their embodied experience and perception of their world, and their means of relating to the Other(s), as pertaining significantly to matters of trust. In synthesising the Husserlian-influenced phenomenology of Schutz and Merleau-Ponty. O'Neill (1972, 1995) seeks to make sociology relevant to the physicality of experiences (such as trust) amidst the social world, and in so doing to transcend the artificial and sanitised data applied by more empiricist social science and medicine – that which censors and absolves research from the meaning of lived experience.

The embodied experience of gynae-cancer: the 'subjective' object of body work
Following this 'turn' towards the body, many more recent sociological accounts are keenly aware of the limitations of medicine in comprehending, and therefore assisting, the experience of the patient: 'for many patients the experience of modern medicine – especially hospital-based medicine – is a disjunctive one, involving not just pain but also dislocation, objectification and a denial of their sense of embodiment' (Twigg 2006: 98). The potential for dislocation, alongside wider issues of subjectivity, are exceedingly apparent within the field of gynaecological oncology – due to the experienced threat of cancer itself, but also due to invasion of the personal/intimate aspects of the female body by strangers such as male surgeons.

The subjective experience of 'illness' cannot be understood outside the diagnosis and treatment enacted by clinicians and the wider abstract system of medicine by which 'patient-hood' is conferred. It is under the spotlight of modern medicine that bodies, especially female bodies, are subject to surveillance (Howson 1998) and where ascriptions of illness (problematisations of the body) create emotional reactions. These responses – within the same body – become important characterisations of the experience of illness (Freund 1998) and are 'lived' in conjunction with the symptoms specific to the pathology. It is in this modern context that 'emotional skills of display, the management of our subjective states, and the "reading" of others' expressions come to be more pervasively used, refined and developed' (Freund 1998: 279) both at a more conscious level but also 'behind one's back'. Such socio-somatic reflexivity not only makes for a pronounced effect of others on self – but furthermore enacts a heightened sensitivity within personal 'imaginative space': 'more "room" to brood, regret, anticipate' (Freund 1998: 280).

If the body is a 'vehicle for being in, experiencing and creating the world in which we live' (Shilling 2005: 69), then the presence of cancer can be understood as a profoundly destabilising attack on the integrity of this existential medium. Such an undermining of 'normal' conceptions of body and thus self through the symbiotic presence of the tumour (Shilling 2008: 124) may manifest itself more immediately – through apparent symptoms (for many of the cervical cancer patients interviewed this was through abnormal discharge or bleeding) – or remotely, as the haunting spectre of the 'battle' which lies ahead (Sontag 1978).

This latter cultural 'baggage', which surrounds the diagnosis of cancer, illustrates the complex and pervasive interlocking between the physical and the social. That an acknowl-edgement of the presence of abnormal cytology is inherently imbued with such significant meaning and socialised assumptions is moreover mirrored in the particular way gynaeco-logical anatomy and functioning are bound up with notions of the feminine self. Impediments to normal sexual and reproductive physical functioning are problematic therefore, as sex is 'not simply what one has, or a static description of what one is: it will be one of the norms by which the "one" becomes viable at all, that which qualifies a body for life within the domain of cultural intelligibility' (Butler 1993: 236).

The indivisibility of the female body from the way experiences (and expectations) of it are structured by the social environment, and the way it in turn shapes experience of the social world (Grosz 1994), ensures that the psycho-social effects of gynaecological abnor-malities represent weighty challenges to the 'ontological security' (the assumptions about the 'continuity of self-identity' and one's place in the world – Giddens 1990:92) of those diagnosed. In this way, prevailing norms within society 'inscribe the subject with a sexually specific and agentically limiting identity' (Shilling 2005: 67). Such identities may thus be acutely undermined by the physiological interruptions of gynaecological cancer (Juraskova *et al.* 2003), where a breakdown in bodily 'order' attests to the tension between 'natural' forces and social norms of 'control' (Williams and Bendelow 1998).

The obstacles posed to the embodied-self are not limited to the cancerous cells however. The intervention designed to remove the tumour and the threat that surrounds it may be similarly problematic for corporal integrity and feminine identity. Whether the intervention is more minor cauterisation of the cervix (LLETZ[2] procedure), surgical (involving removal of tissue which may include removal of the womb), radiotherapy (with short-term side-effects of irradiated skin in the local area) or brachytherapy (the short-term insertion of radioactive 'seeds' via implanted rods) – the body is likely to be irrevocably changed for the better (medical prognosis) *and* the worse (identity). Levine (2007: 45) argues that contemporary societal conceptions propagate notions that 'human bodies are actually designed to function in a loving, empowered way'. Yet the effects of treatment for gynae-cancer may make intimacy problematic, with the experienced removal or dissection of 'femininity' often acting to disempower and disorder.

The phenomena of body work in gynae-oncology: intertwining roles
The preceding section underscores the complex subjectivity of the patient in order to attest to the challenges faced by clinical staff. The work of gynae-oncology professionals thus takes place on two fundamental levels: that which is concerned with the instrumental in terms of physical removal of diseased tissue and treatment of the illness; and the communicative. These latter, 'softer' skills are required to reassure and assist the woman in coming to terms with the interruptions or more permanent disjunctures to notions of self, and to ensure that investigation and treatment are 'neutralised' in terms of gender (i.e. not seen as a male assault on the female body).

The direct encounter with, and performance on, another's body (Gimlin 2007) is the more obvious form of body work. This labour on the body may take place in a number of forms: physical examination (for example, through colposcopy); surgical or other intervention; and post-intervention care work for the woman as an inpatient or at follow-up appointments. Twigg (2000, 2006) describes how the allocation of such roles within medicine is typically prone to a strict, hierarchical division of labour – with the more senior, male staff typically more distanced from intimate contact with, and work on, the body. Yet the case of gynae-oncology represents a notable exception to this general rule. Indeed it is the (often male) consultant or registrar[3], in making the examination/diagnosis, who is likely to be most intimately in contact with the female patient. For whilst many other surgical specialties use distancing technologies for imaging the internal body, the liminality (blurring of borders) between the internal and external involved in this specialty – especially in the case of cervical cancer – engenders a somewhat different set of 'bounded intimacies' (Twigg 2000) to the norm.

In this light it becomes clear that even this more 'instrumental' of functions (examination towards diagnosis) requires significant interpersonal/tactile skills – the tacit *craft* of medicine (Sennett 2008) – as refined by observation, application and practical experience (in contrast to encoded forms disseminated via guidelines[4]). It is within the exercise of this craftwork that apparent dualisms between medical body work as 'paid labour carried out on the bodies of others' and 'the management of embodied emotional experience and display' (Gimlin 2007: 353) begin to break down. Successful examination requires both the ability to inspire trust and facilitate relaxation as much as the dexterous expertise involved in accurately assessing cytology or removing appropriate tissue by biopsy. The art-form, or craft, of 'impression management' (Goffman 1959: 203) – the embodied presentation-of-self in a manner by which the clinician evokes a patient's esteem of their 'character' (Goffman 1959: 244) – is therefore in a number of senses inextricably linked to the more hands-on, intimate and technical body work involved in instrumental diagnosis/interventions.

Trust and intentionality across body work dualisms: spanning form and time
Although the interdependence between 'body work as instrumental contact' and 'body work as performative presentation-of-self' might well be evident in the context of examination, it could be strongly contended that the dualism between the two remains much more sharply defined when surgical interventions are considered (Twigg 2006). Where these are carried out under general anaesthetic, a purely instrumental/technical form of work becomes apparent where no interaction is possible with the unconscious patient. Yet such a mechanical, distanced depiction of this form of body work would ignore two key notions referred to thus far – the 'intentionality' of physical actions, and the trust relations that exist between the surgeon, clinical staff and the patient.

The Husserlian concept of intentionality, as adopted by Merleau-Ponty and Schutz, refers to the importance of meaning for any action. For Schutz (1972: 63), what separates actions from mere unconscious behaviours is the way the former are already 'mapped out' in the 'future perfect tense'. This consideration of future consequences – of a 'projected plan' – is vital for capturing the real meaning of human activity and adds social gravity to the most technical of surgical tasks. In this light, surgical body work becomes far more emotion-laden than it would seem prima facie. For this work does not take place in a chronological vacuum but rather is carried out in anticipation of future consequences when the patient is once again conscious. So whilst to describe the nature of surgical body work as no different from other (consciously interactive) forms would be overly simplistic, the emotion work and moral-relational basis for action remain central.

The *future* consequences of surgery, and the moral obligation based on the relationship formed in the past, thus imbue this activity with far more than is apparent in the immediate present. The heightened awareness of temporality in Schutz's work, following Henri Bergson's considerations of *durée*, also makes evident the increased significance of initial interactions between clinician and patient. Such body work, be it in the form of self-presentation or more touch-involved examination, is not simply effectual on the immediate situation (for example, in easing discomfort or embarrassment at the time of examination). Far more significantly, it is laying the groundwork for a whole legacy of expectations, assumptions, beliefs and hopes which will be drawn on at varying time-points well into the stages of treatment and beyond. These highly complex and multidimensional assurances may more neatly (if somewhat schematically) be referred to under the heading of *trust* – in that the normative obligations laid down by such legacies, alongside wider normative frameworks of professionalism and social interaction, form potent structures within which future action is embedded – thus enabling positive expectations in the light of this structuration (Möllering 2005).

Trust, as noted above, is most straightforwardly conceptualised as expectations which relate to the ability and willingness of the trustee to affect certain outcomes (Calnan and Rowe 2008). Hence, the ability of the professionals to demonstrate that their actions are embedded within norms of competency and care, based on the patient's assumptions as to how these might appear manifest in a clinician, is vital for trust to be won. Regardless of the 'backstage' (Goffman 1959) competency of the clinician (medical knowledge and surgical skill) therefore, their ability to present themselves on the 'front stage' (via various interactions) as competent and caring is decisive in the first instance. Yet the backstage capabilities and motives must also be present if this trust is not to be disappointed. In this sense the pre-intervention, interactive body work (in inducing trust) and the surgical body work (in fulfilling such trust) become inherently bound up with one another – across time – via trust (and the moral obligation it inspires). How body work enables such trust, via the signification of 'latent' or assumed intentionalities, is the concern of the data sections to follow.

The study

The data presented in the following three sections are drawn from semi-structured, qualitative interviews with a sample of 20 women who had recently completed, or were near the end of, their investigation/treatment for cervical cancer. The respondents ranged in age from 28 to 71 and were from a variety of socio-economic backgrounds spanning right across the spectrum, though with a slight overall tendency towards more middle-class brackets. The respondents had experienced a range of 'interventions' – from relatively 'minor' colposcopy examinations with biopsy (as preventative investigation: n = 2) or cauterising procedures (LLETZ[2] as preventative treatment: n = 4), to various combinations of surgery, radio-, chemo- and/or brachytherapy (treatment for cancer: n = 14).

An important limitation of the study is the (white) ethnic homogeneity of the sample. Although 4 of the 20 were white non-British or had spent significant segments of their lives outside Europe, it is likely that the interpretive and embodiment characteristics salient for trust will vary across ethnic groups (Gordon *et al.* 2006). Because of the low presentation of cervical cancer in a small locality (across one NHS acute Trust), all patients who had recently completed or were nearing the end of their treatment were contacted (over a 10-month period). The sample also purposively included those who were involved in screening or preventative measures (see above). The response rate was low (20/61), though perhaps not surprising, given the sensitive nature of the illness experience. Yet the sample included women who reported very high levels of trust, distinctly problematic mistrust, and the more common scenarios by which levels of trust and a poignant awareness of the limitations of trust (and thus anxiety) existed concomitantly.

Following the administration of a short, self-completed quality-of-life questionnaire[5] to grasp a number of potential contextual factors, the interviews typically lasted from 45 to 60 minutes. The interviews were conducted at the home of the interviewee (except for one case at her workplace). Due to the sensitive subject matter respondents were asked if they would like to have a partner/friend sit in on the interviews. This was taken up by three of the respondents and provided some further important insights via the accompaniers' occasional comments. Appropriate ethics clearance was granted by the local NHS ethics committee.

Interviews followed a number of themes seeking to clarify the extent to which trust is dependent on communication by professionals and/or provision of healthcare by the institution (following Brown 2008). The importance of embodied activity for trust was not considered prior to the interviews but became a highly prominent theme within many of the responses. In this sense, the 'open' approach which allowed the 'body work/trust' code to emerge as salient was then followed by more axial coding (Neuman 2000) carried out around this theme, before more selective, cross-case comparisons were made as a further means of expounding theoretical premises. Though thematically-based, the analysis was informed by considerations of the data within the wider biographical and intervention context of each respondent (Coffey and Atkinson, 1996), as well as the immediate experiences of the respondent at the time of interview – as clarified through a quality-of-life questionnaire.

Findings

The following sub-sections describe three characteristics of the embodied phenomenon of trust, as they emerged from the qualitative interview data. First, trust bridged the uncertain present with future expectations (as inferred from prior experiences) and, in so doing, associated different facets of body work with one another. Secondly, the experiential knowledge used to construct trust was dependent on a complementarity of verbal and non-verbal signs. The third sub-section seeks to elucidate further this complex amalgam of signifiers, describing how the verbal often acted to clarify understandings of the mutual agendas on which trust was based, whereas the non-verbal acted significantly to validate these.

Multi-dimensional and multi-temporal body work bearing on trust
As was set out in an earlier section, different facets of body work, as performed by clinicians, function to build trust across a number of temporal 'contexts'. Body work also acts to provide immediate reassurance and to neutralise gender issues, for example, the male consultant is presented as friendly and having the same type of relationship with the patients as do (female) nurses, as the following quotation illustrates:

Sandra[6]:   Yeah, well I felt comfortable enough to be able to joke and chat with him [consultant], and therefore I would have been able to ask him anything. And the nurses, in his clinic, are really nice too, and you can have a laugh and a joke with them. 'Cos to be honest, as you can imagine, you have so many examinations and tests and everything . . . if you didn't have people like that, who you could joke with and humanise yourself, you'd just end up feeling like a piece of meat really.

Here the quality of body work as the presentation of an approachable (unthreatening) self (developed through positive interactions), by which the patient describes being made to feel comfortable, facilitates trust within the more touch-based body work of the examination – ensuring the potential for it to be seen as a male assault is neutralised. The reference to joking emphasises the informality of the relationship but also suggests the use of humour to conceal or deny a possible threatening reality (Giuffre and Williams 2000). The social interaction of the approachable, friendly consultant assures the patient that her body is seen as a locus of attachment to the social world (Shilling 2005), as opposed to mere flesh, and therefore more likely to be cared for within this examination form of body work.

The reference to nurses involves bodywork in two senses. It establishes the consultant as part of a team enabling the relationship with the individual physician to be generalised to the wider abstract system of medicine and professionalism (Giddens 1990). It moreover neutralises the threat to the body presented by the consultant, a male technical expert by associating him with the female 'caring' nurses. This broader, 'humanising' social context is important as trust is facilitated by expectations of shared norms that provide the patient with assurance that the trustee's behaviour is oriented by and embedded within normative obligation (Möllering 2005). Thus, the clinician's body work in the initial consultations can reassure the patient that they share a common purpose and values so that when trust is really needed, for example, during a fateful moment such as surgery under anaesthetic, the patient requires a more modest 'leap of faith' in the agency of the individual.

The reassurance of being able to feel human, even within uncomfortable body work situations, influenced the development of a more general, future-oriented trust in the caring qualities of the clinician. Conversely, the poor body work as touch indicated in the excerpt below was seen as undermining a positive affective disposition towards the doctor in the future:

Jane:	I remember the first time they tried to get the sample it didn't work. And I remember just sort of . . . making a noise when he took this, when it pinched and thinking bloody hell, that was probably worse than I thought it was going to be. And then he [consultant] hadn't done it properly or he hadn't managed to get it, so he had to do it again. So I don't think that really helped his case . . . his place in my heart [laughs].
Interviewer:	And is [your next appointment] with the same chap again?
Jane:	I bloody hope not . . . I'm sure he's very skilled in a way. You just need to put someone at ease the first time you see them.

Hence body work as touch is able to bear on attitudinal positions towards the future (*i.e.* trust).

As argued above, body work as presentation is able to inspire trust in future body work as touch. Below are two responses to a general question as to why a particular consultant surgeon was deemed highly trustworthy – as had been indicated earlier in the interviews. The respondents, both of whom experienced surgical interventions, described their trust as based on quality presentation-of-self:

Rose:	I just think he's just very nice, and he's got a very laid-back attitude, and you feel confident with him [consultant]. I don't know how you exude that from his side, but he does make you feel ok. And that he is going to get round to this and deal with it.
Celia:	Oh, he's great isn't he . . . He's terrific. Totally thorough. I wouldn't say he has a bedside manner. Because I think he's quite shy actually. And he takes it very seriously. And I'm happy with that . . . I had total confidence. Totally. As soon as you meet [this consultant], I think, he has totally got his eye on the ball.

Thus it is the quality of interaction that inspired trust towards the future hands-on interventions. Presumably the characteristics of calmness, seriousness and focus are also associated with those of a capable surgeon. The shyness referred to might furthermore be read as a way of distancing the consultant surgeon from male stereotypes, thus overcoming the potential concerns referred to above regarding a male invasion of the intimate female body.

Importantly, these two somewhat contrasting descriptions (above) refer to the same consultant, thus emphasising the active subjectivity of trust – in terms of which characteristics are deemed important and how these are inferred from the actions of an individual (Brown 2009). Yet the potential for this active 'bracketing' (Sartre 1962) or framing of certain characteristics or temperaments as positive and trustworthy was not equally apparent amongst all respondents. Three respondents had experienced highly negative outcomes from previous interventions (two gynaecological, one obstetric) in their teenage years. The impact of these earlier negative encounters was described as affecting their initial attitudinal position towards their more recent healthcare. One of the three, however, recounted highly positive interactions with certain key clinicians over the course of her treatment – with the quality of this body work as presentation overcoming initial misgivings and facilitating high levels of trust.

In contrast, the other two women described decidedly poor quality presentations-of-self which failed to reassure them. That these were the only two women to describe a problematic lack of trust (amongst the 20 respondents) suggests that negative experiences of body work as touch in the past may be crucial in shaping the interpretation of body work as presentation in the present, and, moreover, how this is applied to construct trust in relation to the future. Unlike the positive inferences drawn from a 'serious' disposition noted earlier, the account below (from one of these two women) illustrates the potential for poor body work as presentation to limit possibilities for trust:

Trudy: . . . they don't have the old-fashioned bedside manner – they're not friendly, it's like it's your fault that they have to work, you're an irritation to them when you go and see them. He [consultant] was sitting in a chair in his office. He didn't get up, didn't shake my hand . . . I didn't warm to him whatsoever.

Complementarity between verbal and non-verbal 'signs'
The previous section noted the way patient interpretations of body work as presentation impact on their experiences of body work as touch – and vice versa – and, furthermore, how these interdependencies function across time. The remaining two sections move on to focus on the form and content of the experiences of body work as presentation. As was indicated in the introduction, trust research has tended to focus on the content of speech acts rather than the actions that make these present and accompany them. The work of Schutz (1972) and other phenomenologists make apparent the importance of both verbal and non-verbal 'signs' which are able to be interpreted in a number of ways. Yet whilst this distinction between content and mode of presentation may be useful analytically, the respondents tended not to make such neat distinctions.

Indeed, much of the data makes apparent the lack of a dualism between style and content, or indeed verbal and non-verbal signs (Hindmarsh and Heath 2000):

Susan: I was really scared to meet doctors . . .
Interviewer: And so were there any things they did to make you trust them or put you at your ease?
Susan: [The GP who made the referral] gets in a flap, he's very real – so he'll let you see that. So he's just himself. If he does something wrong he goes – 'oh, bloody hell' – and it doesn't bother him. So you can see he's not putting on a front, you know, so, he's himself.

As with Rose's comment (see previous section), this account was one of many which described trust as developing out of a complex (sometimes nebulous) amalgam of signs. As indicated in the quotation below, the phenomenon was a communicatively embodied whole. Whilst the overall impression was one of being in control, what generated this was not reducible to any one particular attribute or action:

Caroline: . . . he [consultant] had the whole package if you like . . . [he was] in control . . . so yeah.

Even when specific moments of trust-winning behaviour could be more clearly elucidated, it was evident that these were again intricate weaves of physical movements, verbal interactions and mere temporal presence:

Esther: I heard the buzzer going *constantly* through the night, and I really don't think they have enough manpower at certain times – I'm sure everyone must say that to you mustn't they? And this one on the night when I was really struggling, I mean, she [nurse] was amazing. You wouldn't have thought there was anyone else she was caring for. She just had that knack – you never felt she was rushed, she'd just sit down on the chair next to you.

In this instance, it is the focused attention of the nurse, embodied by her devoting time amidst a busy ward, which is crucial. The system-based pressures on a nurse's time (as inferred from the general work space) ensure that her agency, in spending time with the patient in spite of working structures which would make this difficult, is interpreted as a starker indication of her care for the patient than would be the case in a well staffed ward. So while conducive normative structures (as suggested above) may make attributions of trust more straightforward, communicative agency in spite of obstructive instrumental structures (Brown 2008) also acts to emphasise the power of norms – thus enabling trust. This is achieved through spatial location and physical signs as much as utterances.

The manner by which verbal and non-verbal signs complement one another in developing a more general impression on the patient is evident within the scene described below. Trudy was the patient quoted at the end of the preceding section with very low levels of trust and poor interactive experiences with some of the doctors she was treated by. In contrast, she describes the words and actions of the lymphodemist she saw as part of her treatment:

Trudy: I mean she sat down next to me, she smiled, she took an interest in me, she said to me – 'was there anything else that I can explain for you'. She was just genuinely interested, she didn't rush through anything. I was expecting about a five/ten minute urm, consultant [*sic*] whatever, we were there for half an hour, she wasn't rushed to get out, she gave me a sheet to cover myself with which the other doctor never bothered doing. That kind of thing, she cared for me as a person, she didn't worry about what *she* was doing or rush off to go and do *her* thing [original emphasis].

The way this intricate lattice of signs, verbal and non-verbal, may be bracketed together under a general impression – such as 'trustworthy' – is usefully summed by Crossley (2007: 84), following Merleau-Ponty: 'The other is not a physical thing for me but rather is a locus of meaning. Their posture, comportment, gestures, and movement communicate to me and it is the meaning of such communication which occupies the foreground of my perception. I see and hear happiness or a welcome rather than the physical movements which convey these sentiments'. Thus it is the ability of these manifold signs to resonate meaning – relating to competence and especially an inferred intentionality of care – which enables their trust-invoking capacity.

The significance of physical action – a more concrete basis of 'knowledge' and meaning
The power of verbal and non-verbal actions to signify a more hidden, or latent, intentionality has been seen thus far as central to the building of trust. Indeed, the use of language 'is capable of "making present" a variety of objects that are spatially, temporally and socially absent from the "here and now"' (Berger and Luckmann, 1966:174). Yet if language is powerful, arguably the use of non-verbal signs as a means of indicating trustworthiness is more potent still. For pictures, and actions, can be 'worth a thousand words', as the

saying suggests, through the multi-dimensionality of performance which involves 'manner', 'appearance', 'etiquette' and other such signifiers, and presents these to be interpreted within a certain physical and social 'setting' (Goffman 1959).

To explore this truism a little further, it is the ability of actions to corroborate truth claims of intentions, relating to trustworthiness, which makes them so significant. In the final data excerpt in the previous section the professional not only articulates her considerateness by ensuring the patient understands, but her facial expressions and other actions substantiate these. In stark contrast, one of this patient's less positive encounters highlights how poor presentation-of-self can betray any verbal claim to the contrary:

Trudy: And as I was doing that [getting undressed before the examination] I could hear him [registrar] sitting in his chair yawning as though – 'you're wasting my time'.

Here, the slightest of gestures by a registrar is indeed held to speak a volume of words. Yet this is not to say that words are irrelevant to trust. In the same way that a disembodied portrayal of trust is problematically limited, one which fails to acknowledge the relevance of words is equally compromised. Williams (2007) describes trust as a belief by the truster that the trustee has her best interests at heart and no agenda to the contrary. Often the form and content of this agenda, especially within the complexity of modern medicine, will be clarified through spoken communication. The women interviewed commonly reflected on verbal utterances as being able to offer rocks of certitude within a wider sea of uncertainty:

Claire: The thing I love about [my consultant] is that, you know, he doesn't bullshit you. You walk in, and the first thing he said to me was – 'right, it's not good news. You've got it, and you've got this stage' . . . And he said 'this is our plan of action'.

However, as seen in preceding sections, actions are often vital in fleshing out the validity of these utterances – moving them from mere words to more concrete assumptions that the trustee is willing and able to fulfil this agenda. Schutz (1972) argues, following Husserl, that all knowledge is only accessible through inferences based on direct experiences. Hence, more abstract notions, such as those described merely by words, require a larger number of inferential steps in order to be comprehended and are correspondingly more tentative – or less 'real'. On the other hand, physical actions are more immediately experienced, and therefore do not require provisional inferences – thus making them more concrete (and often more intricate) as a basis of knowledge. The potency of this latter form is evident here:

Caroline: He [registrar] just put me at ease. Just his manner really.
Interviewer: And just to dig a little deeper, what was it about his manner that was good?
Caroline: He was just really helpful, he said – oh, I'll come down with you if you like I'm not too busy. To have the bloods taken. I'll show you where it is, I'll take you down there. So you didn't feel like you were being sent off.

That a busy registrar is willing to take the time to accompany his patient and help her shows a clear prioritisation of an agenda – her wellbeing – above alternative considerations. Whilst it might be taken as a given that the registrar's agenda would be the best for his patient, it was the concreteness of his actions which corroborated this – enabling such an esteem of his 'manner' and therefore character. The power of such action, especially when it was seen as going beyond that which might be typically expected, was deemed to be especially effective at building trust.

Conclusion: the importance of body work for trust

This chapter has underlined the importance of body work for understandings of trust and its development. The theory and data outlined here have emphasised the potency of embodied interactions, and acknowledged the way signs (verbal and non-verbal) are interpreted by patients, to develop assumptions as to the trustworthiness of their clinicians. This interpretative process is very much based on ideal-typical assumptions (Schutz 1972) of how a competent or caring clinician might appear. These stereotypes are formed through prior socio-biographical experiences and hence the ability of the clinician to accurately gauge the socialised expectations of the patient, and 'pitch' their interactive style accordingly, is vital for building trust.

The multi-temporality of trust also sheds light on the interdependent linkages (and liminality) between different types of body work – especially within the sub-specialty of gynae-oncology. Trust, and the affective relationship on which it is based, bridges the present with the future. Furthermore, it makes apparent how some ostensibly 'detached' forms of body work (the non-tactile presentation-of-self or the technical and distanced work of surgery) are inherently connected with both the emotion-work of the caring role and the craftwork of body work as touch. For it is the meaning attached to this work (for both the clinician and patient), which is vital, as much as the actual specificities of the actions. The role of the perceived and experienced body as a locus for shared common experience and understanding thus enables it to 'shape human sensibility, thought and perception' (O'Neill 1972: 159) in a manner which spans different forms of body work across spatial and temporal locations. The body thus becomes a focus of intentionalities (of the patient and professional) which connect past, present and future.

It must be recognised, however, that this study has referred quite exclusively (theoretically and empirically) to the context of gynae-oncology and thus to a particular physiological, emotional, clinical, cultural and gendered context of body work. Trust and the way that it is embodied through presentation-of-self and body work as touch is likely to vary markedly across clinical settings – as the aspects of Lee-Treweek's (2002) study which touch on the embodying of trust in a quite different setting (cranial osteopathy) make apparent. Further research in terms of cross-contextual comparisons would no doubt help to refine understandings of the way in which competencies and motivations might be embodied in different modes across a range of healthcare contexts.

Yet in spite of its particularities, the present study involving cervical cancer patients nonetheless allows some general observations to be made around the importance of embodied interactions with patients. Whereas clear verbal communication is vital in providing semblances of clarity and certainty amidst a wider sea of complexity, practitioners should be keenly aware of the way their presentation-of-self and body work as touch can generate or undermine trust. The smallest of gestures (taking time to draw a sketch by way of anatomical exposition) can have significant positive impacts on trust, through the inferring of intentionality, which in turn attenuates anxiety. Correspondingly, unwitting behaviours (even apparently minor ones such as yawning at inopportune moments) can seriously undermine the potential for trust.

The impact of such individual action must be understood within wider structures. On the side of the patient, their initial attitudinal position – for example, the presence or absence

120   Patrick R. Brown, Andy Alaszewski, Trish Swift and Andy Nordin

of a 'will to trust' – is vital in the way small signs may be focused upon or disregarded (Brown 2009). Similarly, the ability of professionals to carry out emotion-work effectively is facilitated or constrained by the wider institution – the inadvertent yawn may result from, or be taken as evidence of, overworked and under-resourced departments. In this way attributions of trust are decisively dependent on the regulation of action by social structures (Möllering 2005) – with assumptions of trustworthiness based on the trustee's apparent embeddedness within *normative* structures as opposed to purely instrumental ones (Brown 2008). The combining of verbal and physical signs within body work would seem to offer more compelling evidence of this embeddedness, as well as corroborating professional competence.

The instrumentalisation of medicine (Harrison 2009) may, in the short-term at least, make normative structures more visible – for example, a clinician spending extended time with patients elicits trust due to inferences that caring concerns override performativity demands of the system. The durability of such communicative action in winning trust in the longer-term should not be taken for granted and requires further research. As argued here, the embodiedness of clinical interactions are likely to be central to the effective analysis of this phenomenon.

Acknowledgements

The authors would like to thank Tanya Bunsell, Sarah Evans, Chris Shilling, the peer reviewers and the editors of this volume for their valuable insights. We are especially grateful to the women who gave up their time and shared their experiences.

Notes

1   In this sense, one distinct limitation of the study is that the gynae-oncologists treating the respondents in the study were invariably men. While a range of other female professionals was referred to, this chapter is unable to analyse the gendered differences around the intentionality of surgeons in particular. The data did point to the salience of this issue for some respondents however – for example, the view that male doctors ought to demonstrate a respect for the intimacy of gynaecological exams in a different way from what would be the case if the surgeon were a woman.
2   Long Loop Excision of Transition Zone.
3   Consultant is the term used to describe the highest level of qualified doctor in British medicine. Registrar is the next highest level.
4   The National Institute of Health and Clinical Excellence produces highly esteemed guidelines across a wide-range of clinical areas. Yet the encoding of medical practice within such stipulations has been criticised as reducing medicine to a disembodied technical exercise which ignores the craftwork, interaction and anomalous situations common to all medical practice (Nettleton *et al.* 2008, Brown 2008).
5   The questionnaire included the two modules in the EORTC quality of life tool specifically designed for cervical cancer patients – see Greimel *et al.* (2006).
6   All names used have been changed to ensure anonymity in line with ethical considerations.

References

Berger, P. and Luckmann, T. (1966) *The Social Construction of Reality*. London: Penguin.
Brown, P. (2008) Trusting in the new NHS: instrumental versus communicative action, *Sociology of Health and Illness*, 30, 3, 349–63.

Brown, P. (2009) The phenomenology of trust: a Schutzian analysis of the social construction of knowledge by gynae-oncology patients, *Health, Risk and Society*, 11, 5, 391–407.

Brownlie, J., Greene, A. and Howson, A. (2008) *Researching Trust and Health*. London: Routledge.

Butler, J. (1993) Bodies that matter. In Price, J. and Shildrick, M. (eds) *Feminist Theory and the Body: a Reader*. New York: Routledge.

Calnan, M. and Rowe, R. (2008) Trust, accountability and choice, *Health, Risk and Society*, 10, 3, 201–06.

Coffey, A. and Atkinson, P. (1996) *Making Sense of Qualitative Data: Complementary Research Strategies*. London: Sage.

Cohen, F. and Lazarus, R. (1973) Active coping processes, coping dispositions, and recovery from surgery, *Psycho-somatic Medicine*, 35, 375–89.

Crossley, N. (2007) Researching embodiment by way of body techniques. In Shilling, C. (ed.) *Embodying Sociology: Retrospect, Progress and Prospects*. Oxford: Blackwell.

Department of Health (2007) *Trust, Assurance and Safety – the Regulation of Health Professionals in the 21st Century*. London: TSO.

Elliott, A. (2004) *Subject to Ourselves: Social Theory, Psychoanalysis and Postmodernity*. 2nd Edition. Boulder: Paradigm.

Freund, P. (1998) Social performances and their discontents: the biopsychosocial aspects of drama-turgical stress. In Bendelow, G. and Williams, S. (eds) *Emotions in Social Life: Critical Themes and Contemporary Issues*. London: Routledge.

Giddens, A. (1990) *The Consequences of Modernity*. Cambridge: Polity.

Gimlin, D. (2007) What is bodywork? A review of the literature, *Sociology Compass*, 1, 1, 353–70.

Giuffre, P. and Williams, C. (2000) Not just bodies: strategies for desexualising the physical examina-tion of patients, *Gender and Society*, 14, 3, 457–82.

Goffman, E. (1959) *The Presentation of Self in Everyday Life*. Garden City: Doubleday.

Gordon, H., Street, R., Sharf, B., Kelly, P. and Souchek, J. (2006) Racial differences in trust and lung cancer patients' perceptions of physician communication, *Journal of Clinical Oncology*, 24, 6, 904–09.

Greimel, E., Kuljanic Vlasic, K., Waldenstrom, A., Duric, V., Jensen, P., Singer, S., Chie, W., Nordin, A., Bjelic Radisic, V. and Wydra, D. (2006) The European Organization for Research and Treatment of Cancer (EORTC) quality-of-life questionnaire cervical cancer module: EORTC QLQ-CX24, *Cancer*, 107, 1812–22.

Grosz, E. (1994) *Volatile Bodies: Towards a Corporeal Feminism*. Bloomington: Indiana University Press.

Habermas, J. (1987) *Theory of Communicative Action. Volume 2: Lifeworld and System: a Critique of Functionalist Reason*. Cambridge: Polity.

Harrison, S. (2009) Co-option, commodification and the medical mode: governing UK medicine since 1991, *Public Administration*, 87, 2, 184–97.

Harrison, S. and Smith, C. (2004) Trust and moral motivation: redundant resources in health and social care? *Policy and Politics*, 32, 3, 371–86.

Hindmarsh, J. and Heath, C. (2000) Embodied reference: a study of deixis in workplace interaction, *Journal of Pragmatics*, 32, 12, 1855–78.

Howson, A. (1998) Embodied obligation: the female body and health surveillance. In Nettleton, S. and Watson, J. (eds) *The Body in Everyday Life*. London: Routledge.

Juraskova, I., Butow, P., Robertson, R., Sharpe, L., McLeod, C. and Hacker, N. (2003) Post-treatment sexual adjustment following cervical and endometrial cancer: a qualitative insight, *Psycho-Oncology*, 12, 3, 267–79.

Lee-Treweek, G. (2002) Trust in complementary medicine: the case of cranial osteopathy, *Sociological Review*, 50, 1, 48–68.

Levine, D. (2007) Somatic elements in social conflict. In Shilling, C. (ed.) *Embodying Sociology: Retrospect, Progress and Prospects*. Oxford: Blackwell.

Merleau-Ponty, M. (1968) *The Visible and the Invisible*. Evanston: Northwestern University Press.

Möllering, G. (2005) The trust/control duality: an integrative perspective on positive expectations of others, *International Sociology*, 20, 3, 283–305.

Nettleton, S., Burrows, R. and Watt, I. (2008). Regulating medical bodies? The 'modernisation' of the NHS and the disembodiment of clinical knowledge, *Sociology of Health and Illness*, 30, 3, 333–48.

Neuman, W. (2000) *Social Research Methods: Qualitative and Quantitative Approaches*, Boston: Allyn and Bacon.

O'Neill, J. (1972) *Sociology as a Skin Trade*. London: Heinemann.

O'Neill, J. (1995) *The Poverty of Post-Modernity*. London: Routledge.

Poortinga, W. and Pidgeon, N. (2003) Exploring the dimensionality of trust in risk regulation, *Risk Analysis*, 23, 961–73.

Sartre, J-P. (1962) *A Sketch for a Theory of the Emotions*. London: Methuen.

Schutz, A. (1972) *The Phenomenology of the Social World*. London: Heinemann.

Sennett, R. (2008) *The Craftsman*. London: Allen Lane.

Shilling, C. (2005) *The Body in Culture, Technology and Society*. London: Sage.

Shilling, C. (2008) *Changing Bodies: Habit, Crisis and Creativity*. London: Sage.

Sontag, S. (1978) *Illness as Metaphor*. New York: Farrar, Straus and Giroux.

Taylor-Gooby, P. (2008) *Reframing Social Citizenship*. Oxford: Oxford University Press.

Twigg, J. (2000) Carework as a form of bodywork, *Ageing and Society*, 20, 389–411.

Twigg, J. (2006) *The Body in Health and Social Care*. London: Palgrave and Macmillan.

Williams, R. (2007) *Tokens of Trust*. Norwich: Canterbury Press.

Williams, S. and Bendelow, G. (1998) *The Lived Body: Sociological Themes, Embodied Issues*. London: Routledge.

9

Body work in respiratory physiological examinations
Per Måseide

Introduction

The term 'body work' carries different meanings (Shilling 2005, Wolkowitz 2006). In medicine 'body work' refers not only to work in relation to the patient's body but also to corporeal work conducted by healthcare professionals or patients. The body work focused on in this chapter takes place during a certain kind of medical examination. In the past, sociological studies have focused on physical examinations in the medical consulting room (Frankel 1983, Heath 1986). Such examinations have been approached analytically in terms of 'body work' (Heath 2006). The focus has been on doctors' and patients' mutual and practical constitution of bodies as medical objects and tools, while attending to their shared administration of socially, morally and professionally adequate forms of physical contact. Doctors and patients use specific 'techniques of the body' (Mauss 2006), which include the application of gaze in connection with the doctor's physical contact with the patient's body. Emerson (1970) made similar observations of the participants' collaborative efforts to generate and maintain a professionally defined situation during gynecological examinations.

Many medical examinations conducted in hospitals 'belong' to medical specialties, such as radiology, gastroenterology or thoracic medicine; they are conducted at special sites by a doctor or a team of healthcare professionals. Some examinations are ordinarily conducted without attending doctors. Characteristic of such examinations is the centrality of technology. Some examinations are, for instance, conducted by surgeons while the patient is under a general anaesthetic. The body work associated with such examinations is affected by the patient's corporeal condition and is routinely characterised by a restricted professional focus on a pacified and 'objectified' patient body. Other examinations, like bronchoscope examinations, may also have a pacified body as their object, but the framing of the examination is influenced by the fact that the patient is awake and conscious throughout (Måseide forthcoming). In still other examinations an active patient is needed. Cussins (1996) concludes that even if the sense of objectification resulting from a medical examination is experienced by the patient as immediately alienating, it may be positive to the patient's sense of self in the long run.

This chapter considers body work surrounding respiratory physiological examinations conducted in the respiratory physiological lab of a Norwegian hospital ward. The quality of the examinations depended on the correct use of technology and adequate body work

Body Work in Health and Social Care, First Edition. Edited by Julia Twigg, Carol Wolkowitz, Rachel Lara Cohen and Sarah Nettleton.
Chapters © 2011 The Authors. Book compilation © 2011 Foundation for the Sociology of Health & Illness / Blackwell Publishing Ltd. Published 2011 by Blackwell Publishing Ltd.

by professionals and patients. The professionals' body work was not direct hands-on work; their contact with the patient was communicative, informed and was guided by technical devices. The examination aimed at measuring objective physiological respiratory capacities and functions of the patient's body, independent of the patient's volition. To do so, an active and compliant patient was needed. The output of the examination was a textual artefact that in the examination situation counted as the accurate and objective representation of the patient's respiratory physiological status. The examinations represented a mutually constitutive process between various agents, bodies and bodily modes; different kinds of body work were essential for these processes.

Data for the chapter came from an ethnographic study of collaborative medical problem solving in the thoracic ward of a Norwegian teaching hospital. Observations of professional and multi-professional problem-solving activities were conducted during intensive periods of varying length, spread over a period of three years. Throughout this period medical examinations commonly and characteristically conducted in the ward were also observed. Among these were ten respiratory physiological examinations. Because of technical and procedural standardisations they all appeared to be quite similar. Hence, only one examination is presented in this chapter as a case study. Video recordings were not allowed, so data referring to the examinations are based on field notes. The project was approved by the Regional Committee for Medical and Health Research Ethics.

Theoretical framework

In healthcare settings professional work may require hands-on contact with the patient's body. Reading a patient's medical records or filling in a form are other kinds of professional work. Talk and interaction also represent medical work. These forms of work count as body work; they are corporeally conducted and have the patient's body as their direct or indirect object. Since a medical object may be defined by practice and since a patient's body is the object of multiple forms of professional practices and is variously involved in those practices (Mol 2002), the question arises: should the examined patient be described in terms of multiple bodies?

Medical activities may seek to separate body from mind to shape a professionally adapted objective body (Harré 1994, Mol 2002). This objective body belongs to a disciplinary perspective or discourse often referred to as 'the medical model' (Gerhardt 1989). The medical model demands and outlines a specific kind of body particularly designed for medical activities. Other analysts of medical work have described this kind of body as the typical object of biomedical attention and practice (Freidson 1970, Atkinson 1988). In this chapter the term 'objective body' refers to the patient's body in flesh as it is professionally approached in a certain kind of medical examination.

A conceptual distinction informed by Merleau-Ponty (1962) between the 'objective body' and the 'lived body' or 'body-subject' is pursued here for further analysis. The 'objective body' is a physical or biological entity separated from the individual's mind, subjectivity or self. In medicine the objective body may be separated from the social subject through different kinds of separation practices, such as anaesthetics, professional body techniques (Harré 1994), the objectifying 'clinical gaze' (Foucault 1973, Armstrong 1983) and by technology (Bronzino et al. 1990, Atkinson 1995). In contrast to 'the objective body', the terms 'lived body' and 'body-subject' refer to an active, subjective and experiencing body. According to Merleau-Ponty (1962) we are our bodies; our body is our way of being-in-the-world, of participating and practising in this world and it is the centre from which we perceive and experience our world at different times and under different circumstances. The lived body's meaningful practices and experiences are products of interaction with and reflexivity in relation to this body's practical surroundings. We experience and learn to know our bodies by being active in our world (Ihde 2002).

Following from the above characterisations, the patient's 'objective body' is the instrumental object of professional work in the respiratory physiological examinations. But the patient's 'lived body' experiences the examination and conducts the required body work. The lived body is also attended to by the professionals during the examination. In line with Merleau-Ponty's distinction then, the respiratory physiological examinations involve at least two conceptions of bodies, and a certain slippage may exist between them.

The respiratory physiological examinations produce information about the patient's body and its respiratory physiological functions. This information appears in the form of visual images and textual representations that suggest a third kind of body produced by body work. This may be termed the 'virtual body' or 'image body' (Ihde 2002). It is not a body in flesh and not a body-subject. It is an artificial, abstract and restricted body, shaped by technology, professional knowledge and body work. The most proximate purpose of the respiratory physiological examination is to produce a virtual body. In hospital medicine, virtual bodies are vital for the extensive collaborative medical problem-solving work conducted without direct patient contact. This chapter will highlight body work conducted by the patient and the professional to generate and relate adequately to the fluctuating objective, collaborative and virtual bodies surrounding the examination.

Examinations, exactness and body work

A large proportion of the thoracic ward's patients are examined in the respiratory physiological lab. One of the most common diseases diagnosed and monitored is Chronic Obstructive Pulmonary Disease (COPD). Other diseases include asthma, sarcoidosis, pulmonary fibrosis and cystic fibrosis. The examinations are often part of the diagnostic process. They are also used to evaluate a patient's respiratory capacity if surgery is considered and they may be used to monitor the development of a disease or to measure effects of treatment. The examination externalises the body's internal vital functions and turns them into digital and analogue signs with the help of computers and mathematical algorithms. It produces a virtual body precisely designed for further clinical work. When doctors later attend to the patient's respiratory functions, they turn to this virtual body.

The lab accomplishes what the chief physician described as 'the most exact science' in the thoracic ward. The virtues of exactness were also stressed by the professionals working in the lab when they talked about the quality of the technical equipment in use and the results this equipment produced. The equipment was described as very sensitive to changes in environmental conditions, such as temperature and atmospheric pressure and these were constantly tested and calibrated. Doctors and bioengineers also emphasised the necessity of correct and exact testing practices. According to doctors and bioengineers who conducted such examinations, the most common source of failure was not technology; the problem was usually patients who did not follow instructions. Some patients did not understand the instructions or did not use the technical equipment adequately. A few doctors also mentioned that the bioengineers in charge of the examinations did not always do their job properly. One of the residents declared that the validity of data from these examinations depended very much on the work of the bioengineer in charge. Doctors would, for instance, follow the development of a disease like sarcoidosis by regularly running respiratory physiological tests. The test results improved as the patient got better; but sometimes one examination result might unexpectedly deviate from the improving tendency of earlier examinations. Why was that? The answer, the doctor said, depended on who was in charge of the examination. The sudden deviance would most likely be the result of sloppy work by the bioengineer. Some doctors in the ward reported that they did not have the same confidence in all bioengineers and therefore also not in all examination results. The chief physician also emphasised that results from the examinations very much depended on the quality of the bioengineers' work. In turn the bioengineers emphasised that good communication with the patient was essential for correct examinations. The exactness of the examinations was thus not only a product of perfect technology; it was also a product of adequate communication and body work.

A brief description of respiratory physiological examinations

Respiratory physiological examinations or Pulmonary Function Tests (PFT) measure differences in lung volume and lung capacity. 'Lung capacity' refers to lung volume in connection with inhalation and expiration. A bioengineer is usually in charge of the tests, which include the patient's correct inhalation, expiration and use of the measuring equipment. This means that the bioengineer is in charge of the patient's body work. A correct test demands that the patient seals his or her lips tightly around a mouthpiece to inhale and exhale correctly. A clip is fastened to the patient's nose during the test to ensure that no air escapes that way. The tests are repeated several times; institutional procedures determine how many tests should be run. During the tests the patient's inhalation and expiration are visualised on a monitor. The following is a description of the most commonly observed tests in the lab:

- FEV1 (forced expiratory volume in one second) measures the amount of air a person is able to exhale forcefully in one second. What counts as normal results for this test will differ according to the test person's age, height, weight and ethnicity. Information about that has to be fed into the computer. This test is used for diagnosing and monitoring the development of airway obstructions or bronchial constrictions such as asthma or emphysema.
- FVC (forced vital capacity) measures the total amount of air a person can forcefully exhale in one breath after maximal inspiration.
- FEV1/FVC (pulmonary function test) provides a calculated ratio; it shows the proportion of forced amount of air exhaled in the first second of maximal expiration. This test can be used to distinguish between restrictive (i.e. pulmonary fibrosis or sarcoidosis) and obstructive pulmonary diseases (i.e. asthma or COPD).
- PEF (peak flow) measures the speed of air that is forcefully exhaled through the bronchi. This measurement is simple and highly correlated with FEV1.

Two more tests are also common. DLCO (Diffusing Capacity of the Lung for Carbon Monoxide) also termed 'the lung diffusion capacity test' measures the extent to which oxygen passes from the lungs into the blood. The results of this test may indicate various pathological conditions such as COPD, pulmonal fibrosis, emphysema and alveolitis. Another test concerns the measurement of 'residual volume' (RV). 'Residual volume' is the remaining volume of air in the lung when enforced expiration is completed after a full inhalation. The residual volume increases with obstructive pulmonary diseases.

The bodily functions examined in the respiratory physiological lab are not directly observable. They are made measurable, are measured and made observable through the use of technical devices in combination with the patient's body work of inhaling and exhaling. Bioengineers contribute to the production of test results by instructing the patient in how to conduct the necessary body work, by monitoring the patient's body work through direct observation (how the patient manages his or her inhalation, expiration or panting and how he or she uses the technical equipment), and through observations of visual images that represent the patient's respiratory physiological functions. They also make assessments of how the technical equipment works.

Body work and the multiplicity of bodies

All examinations start with a bioengineer recording information about the patient. She (those observed were all female) is seated at a computer, which is connected to the measurement equipment. The patient sits on a chair at her side. Before the examination starts, a mouthpiece for breathing is regulated to fit the patient's body. When the patient has the mouthpiece in his or her mouth, in the words of Ihde (2002), a 'human-technology symbiosis' is established. To conduct the examination the patient's body must be perfectly adapted to the technical equipment. The technology makes the patient's body work in extraordinary ways. The patient may strive to keep the mouthpiece correctly in his or her mouth and to breathe through it in a manner adequate for the examination. If the mouthpiece and the patient's body do not interact correctly, or if the patient does not breathe correctly for the measuring purposes, or if the bioengineer does not observe how the patient performs and does not provide instructions or corrections, or if she does not read the monitors adequately, then incorrect data ensue. Extract 1 concerns the initial part of one observed examination involving a middle-aged male patient. It is a diagnostic examination. Subsequent tests from the same examination are described below:

Extract 1:
The bioengineer asks the patient how tall he is, his weight and date of birth. The patient provides the information as requested. 'Then you have just had a birthday' the bioengineer says. She then asks the patient if he has done breathing tests in the out-patient clinic and how they were. The patient again provides the requested information. 'Have you heavy breathing now?' she asks. The patient answers that it only happens occasionally, if he is exposed to dust. 'I suppose that's why I'm here' he adds. 'I tried to work in a tunnel some time ago, but it didn't work out'. The bioengineer then instructs the patient about how he should breathe during the test. She also tells him that she will give additional information while he breathes. When the test is about to start the bioengineer makes the patient aware that his mouth does not close tightly enough around the mouth-piece and she tells him how to do it correctly. Then the test starts.

Before the test starts, significant information about the patient's sex, height, weight and age is registered and stored in the computer. This is information about the objective body to be tested. But a body-subject is addressed to provide such information. When the bioengineer hears the patient's date of birth, she makes a remark about his recent birthday. This marks a departure from the examination script. Implicitly, a change of membership categorisation is made as the bioengineer, for a moment, leaves her professional concern with the patient's objective body and addresses the patient as a member of a shared everyday world. She thus establishes, for the moment, an institutionally irrelevant 'situational co-membership' (Erickson and Shultz 1982). Communicative moves like these are called 'footing' (Goffman 1981). They lead to change of alignment taken to one self or to the other. By her remark the bioengineer involves the patient in the examination as a social subject and 'humanises' the institutional framing of the situation. However, the bioengineer returns quickly to her professional tasks and to the patient's institutional status. She asks if he has done breathing tests earlier. This inquiry is directed to the patient as an experiencing body-subject; it is relevant for the patient's body work during the examination. She also asks about the quality of his breathing today. Such information about the patient's objective body is significant for evaluation of the results of his body work during the examination. The patient is then informed about how to inhale and exhale during the test. This is also information directed to a body-subject. When the patient does not close his mouth correctly around the mouth piece, the bioengineer instructs him how to do it. So the patient as a subjective self and the bioengineer (as a subjective self) collaboratively design an objective body which is suitably available for the examination. The instruction is rather direct. A wall chart that visualises how to breathe during the examination is also shown to the patient. Then the test starts (Extract 2)[1].

Extract 2:
Bioengineer: Just sit closer to the mouthpiece and I will adjust the height. I will explain how you will do this. First you will breathe quite normally. After a while you will inhale till I say you should exhale and you will do that as long as I say so. We shall now put on the nose clip. (The nose clip is put on.) Now you just sit there and breathe normally (pause). Inhale COMPLETELY as much as you can, and OUT again ALL you can do, *OUT OUT OUT* and normally. Was it heavy?
Patient: No but I could have been a bit faster when inhaling.
Bioengineer: Yes I can see that, but we will try to make it next time. Breathe normally. Close the mouth tightly around the mouthpiece so you don't let in air. Inhale COMPLETELY, *FULL SPEED OUT*, a bit more, a bit more, a bit more, inhale full speed again, nice! Yes they are quite similar these two (she looks at the monitor where a second curve goes exactly over the first). Breathe normally. Inhale COMPLETELY, full speed OUT again, a little bit more, a bit more, and then inhale again, oh come on!

Extract 2 describes body work. The patient's body and the technical equipment must work as one system; this human-technology symbiosis constitutes what Hirschauer (1991) has called a 'mega organism'. The patient's body, expanded by technology, is a fourth kind of body typical of the respiratory physiological examination. The technical equipment makes demands on the body's physiological functions during the tests. It contributes essentially to the shaping of the body at work. If we follow Ihde's (1990) phenomenological approach, using and adapting to the technical equipment contributes to the patient's corporeal experience of his or her body, and such an experience or sensing is necessary for the patient to accomplish body work mindfully and adequately during the examination. The concrete experience of the equipment, of its materiality, affects the patient's embodied conception of how to use this equipment, which again will have an effect on his breathing.

When instructed on how to accomplish the physical work of the test, the patient is addressed by the bioengineer as a '*you*'. The use of the personal pronoun integrates the patient as a body-subject in the institutional efforts at generating a correct measure of the physical qualities of his objective body. The test starts and the bioengineer commands the patient about what to do and how to do it. This is the bioengineer's body work. It is closely adjusted to that of the patient and it is specifically indexed by her loudness of voice and fastness of speech. She responds verbally to her direct observations of the patient's efforts at adequate body work and to its visual representation on her monitor. Her talking and shouting encourages the patient's efforts. After the first test the bioengineer asks the patient if the work was hard. The patient's response is self-critical. He suggests he might have done better. He might have been in better command of his body during the test. This evaluation of the body work conducted is an exchange between two social subjects. They do not talk about an objective body but about the experiencing subject in command of the body. The bioengineer agrees, but she adds, 'we will try to make it next time'. Her use of plural 'we' indicates that the test results are a joint accomplishment and she shares responsibility for them. It is collaborative body work that produces information about the objective body. A new test is then conducted with approximately the same result as the first. At the end of Extract 2, some talk between the bioengineer and the patient followed. They agreed that the patient had some problems breathing correctly and he admitted that he had smoked a cigarette just before the test. Both breathing technique and cigarette smoking (ideally the patient should not smoke for 24 hours before the examination) affect the patient's performance. There may be a moral element to this confession that should not be restricted to smoking. The patient's admission that he did not perform his best during the test and did not have the situationally required control of his body is normatively significant. It implies that he was not up to the standards of 'what one should be able to do' in situations like this. For the purposes of the examination, optimal body work is medically significant as only this provides correct images of the objective body; but the patient's moral identity or social standing as one who is able to accomplish what is required is also at stake during the examination. This moral dimension is closely related to a phenomenological or pragmatic notion of normativity (Dreyfus 1991: 151–52). It is not grounded in moral principles; it follows instead from a general request for ordinariness. It is the request for ordinary physical capability, for efforts demanded for a specific situation or activity and for the ability to use some piece of equipment adequately.

The next test was the diffusion test (extract 3) and the patient was told to pant. The bioengineer explained that when he pants he will not get enough air, so he will quickly feel that he is 'hitting the wall'. But, the bioengineer assures him, this is as it should be. Before the test starts she repeats the information about correct body techniques for the test.

Extract 3:
Bioengineer: Breathe normally. PANT! (for about seven seconds).
              Breathe normally. Exhale! Inhale again! Breathe normally.

After the first attempt the bioengineer declares that the test failed. They have to repeat it. The patient complains about the nose clip as it lets air through his nose. He has not failed, the equipment is the problem. He is given a new clip and new tests are conducted. The bioengineer explains that the first test was poor not only because of the problem with the nose clip, but also because the patient did not pant as he should and he inhaled too deeply. The latter point implies moral criticism, the patient's body work was not adequately conducted.

When the bioengineer instructs the patient about his body work and urges him during the tests, she uses her voice and body. Her use of hands and arms is particularly vital during the residual volume test. She makes fast movements up and down with her arms to visualise the required speed of the patient's panting and she changes to long and slow arm movements to indicate normal exhalation and inhalation. She holds one of her hands down when he exhales and up when he inhales.

During the tests the bioengineer attends to different kinds of bodies. She addresses the patient as a body-subject; she observes the patient's breathing and panting body and on her monitor she observes the recorded images of this body work. From observing the patient's virtual body she makes assessments of the objective body and the efforts of the body-subject. But her attentiveness is also embodied. She engages corporeally to make the patient do adequate body work. When the bioengineer and the patient talk about the examination after the test has been conducted, a shift of perspective takes place. They talk about the objective body that may not be correctly measured, the body-subject that does not achieve and the virtual body of the monitor that documents the failing achievement. Hence, the patient is involved as body-subject in a double sense. The test results indicate a lived body that does not achieve, and the objective body registered is a product of the body-subject's failing achievement. Responding to this, the patient acts as a subject that tries to achieve and regrets his failing achievement. Achievement is important not only for documenting objective physiological capacity. It also documents the patient's subjective or moral character as achiever. The bioengineer cannot make clinical evaluations of the patient's achievements. The efforts she criticises or praises relate to expectations of a standardised version of the patient's body and his demonstrated will and ability to achieve.

The various kinds of bodies involved in or produced by the examinations are results of the body work conducted by the participants. They are addressed as bodies, social subjects and representations. They also enact objective bodies and body-subjects. They are all parts and products of the examination procedures. They belong to an institutionalised activity and may be described in terms of 'membership categories' (Sacks 1972). These categories are basically of two kinds. On the one hand, they are institutionally embedded and refer to patients, professionals, and the objective or virtual bodies focused on and shaped by technology and institutionalised body work. The institutionalised body work is supposed to generate an institutionally adequate body together with objective and accurate measurements of respiratory physiological functions. On the other hand, they are communicative and refer to the body-subjects or social subjects involved in the examination. The communicative element of body work may in certain respects deviate from institutionalised body work, while it remains integrated within the institutionalised activities and connected to the institutional categories. The distinction between these categories is not made to emphasise the identity work patients may be involved in during medical examinations. The main purpose is to highlight the complexities of bodies and body work characterising respiratory physiological examinations.

Discussion

Ian Hacking (1999) introduced a distinction between 'indifferent' and 'interactive' kinds. 'Kinds' are understood as general or abstract categories. Indifferent kinds refer to what cannot be addressed symbolically as it does not respond to meaning. The concept replaces the commonly used notion of 'natural kind' and defines indirectly the concept of 'interactive kind'. Contrary to indifferent kinds interactive kinds are affected by and function through interpretation and transfer of meaning. The objective body that is tested and measured in the respiratory physiological lab should, according to strict principles of what the examination is supposed to measure, belong to the indifferent kinds. The aim of the examination is to produce an exact measure of what this objective body, for purely biological reasons, is capable of achieving, independent of the patient's volition and other external circumstances. But the body that is measured is also the body that conducts the tests, and the conducting body is a body-subject. Body-subjects belong to the 'interactive kinds'.

The human-technology symbiosis constituted by the patient connected to the measurement equipment is also of an interactive kind. The technical equipment does what it is supposed to do only in adequate interaction with a conscious and mindful patient, who is able to adapt corporeally to the requirements of the technical equipment and the procedural demands of the bioengineer. The results of the tests constitute a virtual body; and even if the virtual body is a material product in the form of a text or of other images that should guide and not be manipulated by the clinician, it also belongs to the interactive kinds. The test results are 'active texts' (Smith 1993), they have an impact, but only when their practical clinical meaning is determined by a physician's reading and re-contextualisation of the text. The significance of any text depends on its status as 'text-as-read', and reading a text means its re-contextualisation (Watson 2009).

This re-contextualisation implies relating test results to the assumed body work of the participants, with a particular focus on the bioengineer in charge of the tests. It also means evaluating the test results in relation to other clinical data, to expectancies and to the practical significance it may or may not have. The virtual body is of an interactive kind also in the sense that it is the product of a body-subject's conscious efforts at achieving optimally and adequately in accordance with the instrumental and normative claims of the situation, the demands of the measuring equipment and the information, instructions and enforcement provided by the bioengineer. It even depends on the bioengineer's accurate observations and interpretations of the patient's efforts and the practical adequacy of her corporeal responses to what she observes.

This analytical concept of 'kinds' may initiate a process of analytical reasoning about bodies, but it may also provide an image of multiple or different bodies. The extent to which Annemarie Mol's (2002) distinction between differently enacted kinds of disease implying a possible distinction between different kinds of bodies is a bit unclear. However, in respiratory physiological examinations only one physical body is examined. To maintain a naturalist and realist perspective on the examination of one body while we recognise the multiplicity hinted at above, we may introduce the term 'body complex'. The term 'kind' that suggests ontological differences, may be substituted by the term 'mode'. The latter refers to a particular form or variety of 'something', a 'core element' exists, which in this case is the individual body. A body may have multiple appearances, functions and meanings, but they all refer and testify to one particular body.

So what appears during the respiratory physiological examinations is a body complex consisting of diverse and, to some extent (but not completely), simultaneous bodily modes. These modes are highlighted, made manifest or suggested at different moments of the examinations. They are products of different types of body work; they are differently displayed and made relevant for different purposes. The body complex referred to is not a natural phenomenon disclosed by the examination, neither is it a multiplicity of bodies. It is an intricate and situational product of interactive practices that differentiates the body into various modes. The term 'bodily modes' suggests unity, complexity and multiplicity of meanings and functions, but not multiplicity of kinds.

With regard to the 'exactness' associated with these examinations, exact measures are not solely technological products, they require collaborative body work, whether the collaboration is between human actors, humans and technology or between humans and texts. Because of this, 'exactness' also belongs to the interactive kinds. It is interactively and situationally produced and it may be re-contextualised and change meaning depending on the setting and the activity it is involved in.

Conclusion

The 'exactness' produced in respiratory physiological examinations requires technical equipment, but this equipment represents what Wertsch (1991) calls 'mediating means'. To produce medical meanings or facts technology must be part of a wider productive system. This system may best be described in terms of collaborative body work and human-technology symbiosis. This productive system produces a body complex consisting of various bodily modes, they are all interactive and cannot represent or produce the kind of 'exactness' that scientific or technological medicine might ask for. In a pragmatic clinical perspective, however, its product may represent a workable standard.

The concepts of 'body complex' and 'bodily modes' suggest a unitary and dynamic approach to understanding bodies in various situations, involved in various activities and displaying various meanings, without virtually compartmentalising the body or transforming the body or its parts or functions into a multiplicity of kinds. It is not transformation of the body that takes place during respiratory physiological examinations, it is transformation of meanings and appearances. Body work is at the heart of these transformations.

An emphasis on the patient as a body-subject may be associated with social identities and identity work. This is not a central topic for this chapter. Instead, collaboration, communication, morality and normativity have been alluded to. The body work of respiratory physiological examinations is not regulated and motivated by technical and medical imperatives alone. It is interpersonally regulated and regulated by a morality of effort. While bioengineers conduct everyday routine work, they deliberately produce objective, virtual bodily modes in collaboration with the patients.

Note

1   Transcription conventions for the extract:

!	Rising voice.
?	Inquiring tone
CAP	Loud talk
CAP	Loud and fast talk

References

Armstrong, D. (1983) *Political Anatomy of the Body: Medical Knowledge in Britain in the Twentieth Century*. Cambridge: Cambridge University Press.
Atkinson, P. (1988) Discourse, descriptions and diagnoses: reproducing normal medicine. In Lock, M. and Gordon, D. (eds) *Biomedicine Examined*. London: Kluwer Academic Publishers.
Atkinson, P. (1995) *Medical Talk and Medical Work: the Liturgy of the Clinic*. London: Sage.
Bronzino, J.D., Smith, V.H. and Wade, M.L. (1990) *Medical Technology and Society: an Interdisciplinary Perspective*. Cambridge MA: MIT Press.

Cussins, C. (1996) Ontological choreography: agency through objectification in infertility clinics, *Social Studies of Science*, 26, 575–610.

Dreyfus, H.L. (1991) *Being-in-the-world: a Commentary on Heidegger's Being and Time, Division 1*. Cambridge MA: The MIT Press.

Emerson, J. (1970) Behaviour in private places: sustaining definitions of reality in gynaecological examinations. In Dreitzel, H.P. (ed.) *Recent Sociology No 2: Patterns of Communicative Behavior*. New York: Macmillan.

Erickson, F. and Shultz, J. (1982) *The Counselor as Gate Keeper: Social Interaction in Interviews*. New York: Academic Press.

Frankel, R.M. (1983) The laying on of hands: aspects of the organization of gaze, touch and talk in medical encounter. In Fisher, S. and Todd, A.D. (eds), *The Social Organization of Doctor-Patient Communication*. Washington DC: Center for Applied Linguistics.

Freidson, E. (1970) *Professional Dominance: the Social Structure of Medical Care*. Chicago: Aldine.

Foucault, M. (1973) *The Birth of the Clinic: an Archeology of Medical Perception*. London: Tavistock.

Gerhardt, U. (1989) *Ideas about Illness: an Intellectual and Political History of Medical Sociology*. London: Macmillan.

Goffman, E. (1981) *Forms of Talk*. Philadelphia: University of Pennsylvania Press.

Hacking, I. (1999) *The Social Construction of What?* Cambridge MA: Harvard University Press.

Harré, R. (1994) *Physical Being: a Theory for Corporeal Psychology*. Oxford: Blackwell.

Heath, C. (1986) *Body Movement and Speech in Medical Interaction*. Cambridge: Cambridge University Press.

Heath, C. (2006) Body work: the collaborative production of the clinical object. In Heritage, J. and Maynard, D.W. (eds) *Communication in Medical Care: Interaction between Primary Care Physicians and Patients*. Cambridge: Cambridge University Press.

Hirschauer, S. (1991) The manufacture of bodies in surgery, *Social Studies of Science*, 21, 279–319.

Ihde, D. (1990) *Technology and the Lifeworld: from Garden to Earth*. Bloomington/Indianapolis: Indiana University Press.

Ihde, D. (2002) *Bodies in Technology*. Minneapolis/London: University of Minnesota Press.

Mauss, M. (2006) *Techniques, Technology and Civilization*. Schlanger, N. (ed.) New York/Oxford: Durkheim Press/Berghahn Books.

Merleau-Ponty, M. (1962) *Phenomenology of Perception*. London: Routledge and Kegan Paul.

Mol, A. (2002) *The Body Multiple: Ontology in Medical Practice*. Durham/London: Duke University Press.

Måseide, P. (forthcoming) The discourse of medical examinations in hospital settings. In Candlin, C. and Sarangi, S. (eds) *Handbook of Communication in Organisations and Professions*. Berlin/New York: Mouton de Gruyter.

Sacks, H. (1972) An initial investigation of the usability of conversational data for doing sociology. In Sudnow, D. (ed.) *Studies in Social Interaction*. New York: Free Press.

Shilling, C. (2005) *The Body in Culture, Technology and Society*. London: Sage.

Smith, D.E. (1993) *Texts, Facts, and Femininity: Exploring the Relations of Ruling*, London: Routledge.

Strauss, A., Fagerhaugh, S., Suczec, B. and Wiener, C. (1982) Sentimental work in the technologized hospital, *Sociology of Health and illness*, 4, 254–78.

Watson, R. (2009) *Analysing Practical and Professional Texts: A Naturalistic Approach*. Farnham: Ashgate.

Wertsch, J.V. (1991) *Voices of the Mind: a Sociocultural Approach to Mediated Action*, London: Harvester Wheatsheaf.

Wolkowitz, C. (2006) *Bodies at Work*. London: Sage.

10

In a moment of mismatch: overseas doctors' adjustments in new hospital environments
Anna Harris

Introduction

I believed that obstetrics is the same all over the world and so I thought that this is certain knowledge that you put in your suitcase and transfer into every country but it is not exactly the same . . .

(Dr Mladen Mück, research participant) (Harris 2009)

[Overseas doctors] are like musicians – using the same instruments – to play a different song.

(Dr. Nikolai Nagorsky, research participant) (Harris 2009)

Doctors are on the move, with their suitcases of instruments and foreign musical repertoires, to work in hospitals around the world. Their migration seems to have captured mainly the attention of demographers, economists and medical educationalists rather than the imagination of sociologists. Yet the ways in which these overseas doctors shift their work practices across contexts should be of considerable sociological interest. There is a significant gap in our understanding not only of doctors' but also of all skilled migrants' processes of learning and knowledge transfer (Williams and Baláž 2008). Related to this, there is very little written about the phenomenological and sensory nature of work (Wolkowitz 2006: 16). This chapter contributes to these areas and to this book on body work, by exploring one doctor's work involving her body and, by extension, an everyday tool. It considers what a contextual shift may reveal about the nature of bodily adjustment at work.

The chapter draws from an ethnographic study of overseas doctors working in Australian hospitals (Harris 2009). In this larger body of research it is argued that overseas doctors negotiate a multifarious (human and non-human) environment through various modes of adjustment. It argues that overseas doctors adjust principally through a process of *situated, embodied, sensory learning*, continually oscillating between their past and the present. This chapter examines the *tactile* dimension of this bodily adjustment, an under-examined area

Body Work in Health and Social Care, First Edition. Edited by Julia Twigg, Carol Wolkowitz, Rachel Lara Cohen and Sarah Nettleton.
Chapters © 2011 The Authors. Book compilation © 2011 Foundation for the Sociology of Health & Illness / Blackwell Publishing Ltd. Published 2011 by Blackwell Publishing Ltd.

of research in health sociology (Moreira 2006: 81), touch being a less privileged sense in most social research more generally (Ingold 2004: 330).

One of the reasons that tactility has been little studied in the social sciences lies in the difficulties of its observation, articulation and written description. Touch is an important part of our habitual and unreflective bodily practice, one of the 'unregistered dimensions of social life' (Conradson 2003: 1984). It is a challenge to analyse the 'unregistered' aspects of research participants' lives. Consequently, in this chapter I use one of *my own* experiences as an overseas doctor. This autoethnographic methodology entails drawing upon sensory recollections of a significant moment in my medical career overseas. Others have undertaken similar processes of personal recollection in medical sociology (*e.g.* Rier 2000) and sociology more broadly (*e.g.* O'Connor 2007, Bartleet 2009). Autoethnographic reflexivity has long been central to the ethnographic enterprise (Atkinson 2006: 400), and it is now increasingly acceptable for sociologists to draw upon their own experience in their work. By using their body as 'an instrument of research' (Paterson 2009: 771), the sociologist can address the call for analytic work that places the body more centrally (Hindmarsh and Pilnick 2007: 1412). Autoethnography can provide what Mildred Baxter (2009: 765) refers to as 'practical lessons in the interaction between theory and experience'. By 'acting as my own informant' (Rapport 1995: 269), I have elucidated fine sensory details of procedural skill that were absent from fieldwork observations and interviews with the overseas doctors in the larger study. Whilst many of the theorists drawn upon in this chapter have similarly used music and/or their own playing of a musical instrument to illustrate the minutiae of bodily adjustment (Tim Ingold, Richard Sennett, Michael Polanyi, Pierre Bourdieu), this chapter suggests that there is a depth of understanding to be found in studies of medical practice too.

Bodily adjustment is difficult to study for another reason, related to its 'unregistered' qualities. In familiar environments, gestures, movements, everyday practices, *alter tacitly*, at a level below our awareness. We are largely unaware of how our own habits change and rarely reconstruct the process by which we achieve skilful practice (Herzfeld 2009: 145). Several have theorised processes of bodily learning in their research, such as Chris Shilling (2007), who studies what he refers to as 'body pedagogics', a term describing the means through which one learns techniques, skills and dispositions, the embodied experiences of acquiring or failing to acquire these skills, and the embodied changes that result. Similarly, Howard Becker (1970) has analysed 'situational adjustment', which he describes as concerning learning the requirements of a situation in order to continue in it and succeed. Becker (1970: 283) believes that both the situation and the person need to be taken into account in such analysis, and that it is when things do not go according to plan, when one does not adjust appropriately, that we find our most interesting cases for analysis.

This chapter contributes to this field of research by emphasising not only the *tactile minutiae* of mundane medical practices, but also the moments of *mismatch*, when action is disrupted. It is in such moments that I suggest we learn something about how our work practices alter and change across contexts. As Becker has also argued, it is when things do not go according to plan that we are made more aware of the steps that have previously faded from consciousness, and thus find an interesting situation for analysis. Rather than focus on the smooth transition of skilled development, I suggest that to more closely examine bodily adjustment we should turn to those who find themselves in *unfamiliar* environments, to 'newcomers' (Lave and Wenger 1994), who make their adjustments *more obviously* because their habitual practice is disrupted. This is the central premise of this chapter in which I argue that by studying *overseas* doctors' bodily adjustment, during moments of mismatch, we learn something about the multifarious environment of their habitual past and about the new environment they find themselves in at that moment. As these are revealed during the interruption, and the cascading events that follow, we also learn something about the nature of how we adjust to the unexpected.

The structure of the chapter proceeds as follows. Initially it outlines how medical learning has historically been recognised as concerning tacit, bodily knowing. These ingrained practices, learnt in particular contexts, extend to include the tools that doctors use everyday, with these instruments very much part of their embodied practice. From these assumptions, the chapter then discusses how an ingrained procedure (intravenous cannula insertion), one in which tools had become almost natural extensions of my hand in a familiar context, became disjointed when I encountered minute differences in equipment in a different country; when I did not follow the equipment's 'script'. In this moment of mismatch, differences were revealed across contexts and I engaged in a process of adjustment that was bodily and environmentally situated. The chapter then extends the work of Maurice Merleau-Ponty, Tim Ingold and Pierre Bourdieu by highlighting what a moment of mismatch – an event to which all three theorists give minimal attention – reveals about bodily adjustment more broadly. To do so, I incorporate Merleau-Ponty's work regarding the layered body, to help flesh out how doctors oscillate between the past and present in moments of adjustment. Finally the chapter examines what this reveals about the overseas doctors' pasts, and about the new environments they find themselves in, before concluding with a discussion of broader implications and areas of future research.

On inserting a cannula

When I finished my internship in Australia I went to work as a locum doctor in a small cottage hospital at the edge of Royal Oak forest, on the outskirts of a village in the west of England. At the end of my shift, at the end of my first week in the hospital, I was asked by a nurse to insert a cannula (see Figure 1) before going home. There were no other doctors in the hospital, and none of the nurses on duty were experienced in cannulation. I did not hesitate to start preparing for this simple task.

Cannulation involves the insertion of a tube into the body for the delivery or removal of fluids, with the aid of a sharp metal introducer. Intravenous cannulation is one of the most common forms of cannulation in hospitals. With gentle traction on the skin with one hand, the cannula is inserted with the clinician's other hand, so that it pierces the patient's skin and then the vein. Once there has been a 'flashback' of blood into the hub of the

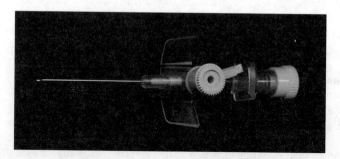

Figure 1 *Intravenous cannula of brand Venflon (manufactured by BD/Becton Dickinson Infusion Therapy AB). 20G (1.0 × 32 mm). Sold in the UK. Photo by Fifo, taken in 2006*

cannula, the flexible tube is inserted a few millimeters further beyond the introducer to ensure proper placement in the vein's lumen. The tube is then fully inserted whilst the introducer is removed and disposed of in a sharps bin. The cannula is 'flushed' with normal saline, capped and taped securely in place. This routine procedure is performed by both doctors and nurses, though in this case it is discussed as the work of a doctor. Thus, rather than the diagnostic or 'high-tech' procedural work that is often emphasised in relation to doctors (Twigg 2000: 390), this chapter focuses on a mundane aspect of medical practice.

Medical touch

It is the feel of the patient's vein that is important when inserting a cannula, for it to happen as quickly and painlessly as possible for the patient. By pressing lightly you can assess how large the vessel is and whether it will stay in place or slip and slide at the whisper of an instrument. Touching happens first without gloves, so that the tactile receptors in the fingertips can judge the depth and pressure required for the introducer to puncture the vein hidden under the skin. Soft bounce, bounce; then quickly on with gloves: quickly, so that your fingers do not forget what the vessel felt like.

When I looked for a place to insert the cannula, when I assessed the patient's veins, I was using my fingertips, intradermally rich in sensory nerve endings, to feel, to touch her skin. Touch has been an implicit part of biomedical practice for some time, with historians recording its importance since the era of humoral medicine, as part of practices such as taking the pulse and palpation (Nutton 1993). Others have discussed the relevance of touch in medicine in contemporary times, particularly in the field of surgery (Pope 2002, Moreira 2006). In many ways the physician's hands are considered 'tools' in their own right. Michael Polanyi (1966: 15) asserts the centrality of the body to the performance of skills, considering it the 'ultimate instrument'.

In many ways, touch is a transportable aspect of 'doctoring', part of a physician's repertoire of embodied practice. Whilst there are numerous cultural nuances regarding touching as part of the clinical encounter, when it comes to procedural work, overseas doctors largely consider the skills ingrained in their hands to be easily transferable (Harris 2009). But clinical touch no longer concerns only flesh-to-flesh contact between the doctor's hands and the patient's body. Since the 19th century, following concern about the bias inherent in tactile medicine, tools have become a common part of medical work. Many historians lament that technology replaced touch, that the two became separated (Reiser 1993: 62, Howes 1995: 130). However, as I argue next, tools are very much part of the embodied work of clinical touch. It is for this reason, that when material differences in equipment are found in an unfamiliar environment, those perceived transportable skills can suddenly fall apart.

Tactile tools

If there was one ingrained procedure during my year as an intern, it was cannula insertion. The cannula had become a natural extension of my hand, cannulation a skill I had learnt, like all interns, to perfect quickly so as to make the job easier. It had become 'second nature' to be able to find a 'good vein' and I had spent my internship sizing up the veins of my friends outside the hospital which bulged in comparison to the patients'.

The technique of cannulation is not learnt by reading and memorising written instructions or by studying illustrations. It is learnt through bodily practice. I started learning cannulation in wetlabs at university, on sections of pigskin, with well-used instruments. Later, as medical students, we practised on each other, leaving tutorials with bruises and dressings. In this practice our hands learnt what other bodies felt like and we got used to the equipment. It was not until we reached the wards however that our bodily learning truly developed during our fleshy-technological interactions with patients. Our hands started to remember these situations, to develop a 'historical density' (Merleau-Ponty 1945: 277). We were taught by interns but it was mostly through practice that we developed our technique, skills honed through repeated trials. The learning curve increased exponentially when we became interns ourselves, and cannulation became a routine activity, always waiting at the end of a paged message or bleep.

The cannula device became an extension of myself during internship, a part of my tacit knowing in the hospital. Polanyi (1966: 16) writes that we make objects function at the proximal end of tacit knowing, that they are incorporated into our body, that we extend our body to include them, 'so that we come to dwell in [them]'. Similarly, Ingold (1996: 179) writes 'in the flow of action, the body itself becomes transparent, as do the tools attached to it'. Ingold draws from Merleau-Ponty who regards instruments as absorbed into the body. Merleau-Ponty (1945: 165) suggests that just as a blind man's stick becomes an area of sensitivity, extending his radius of touch, so 'a woman may, without any calculation, keep a safe distance between the feather in her hat and things which might break it off. She feels where the feather is just as we feel where our hand is'. The feather in the hat is no longer an object but an extension of the woman's body. Objects as such become incorporated into the body, become 'bodily auxiliaries' in familiar settings of practice (Merleau-Ponty 1945: 176). The tools then do not replace touch but rather doctors develop an alternative sense of touch through/with the instruments (Zetka 2003: 18).

A moment of mismatch

In the Nightingale-style ward in that cottage hospital, the patient was sitting in her chair, next to the bed. After briefly introducing myself I rolled out the equipment trolley from the store room. When I started preparing the tools for the procedure I soon realised however that they were different from what I was used to. I was not expecting this. I thought the British system and the Australian system were going to be the same. The difference in the equipment was not large; in fact quite minute. Somehow the instrument did not move as the Australian device I was used to; there was a slight catch as the tubing moved over the introducer.

It meant that on my first attempt of inserting the cannula in the patient's vein, near her wrist, it did not work smoothly. Pulling the patient's tissue paper skin taught, I pierced the epidermis. Jagged and clumsy, then – pop! – into the vein. But because of the arhythmic motion, the introducer went straight through the vessel and out the other side. A slow blue cloud appeared under the patient's skin. The skill I had previously performed fluidly, of entering the vein at the 'right' (not 90 degree) angle, with small shallow angular change milliseconds later so that the pointy introducer did not pierce the other side of the vessel, was suddenly incongruent. The bruise slowly seeped and my pulse rate increased.

When I attempted another insertion, this time near the patient's elbow, I missed again, bursting the vein once more. She looked at me then, in a concerned way – one miss is perhaps forgivable, but not two. The patient said nothing but her eyes asked: 'Does this girl know what she is doing? Where is she from anyway? She doesn't have a British accent. Why did she take so long to assemble the equipment? Did she not know where everything was?'

In this moment of mismatch I was like a piano player who pays attention to their fingers whilst they are playing a difficult piece, gets confused and has to stop (Polanyi 1966: 56). I became conscious of a procedure that I had normally been unaware of, that had been habitual. What had previously been a smoothly embodied action became disjointed when the equipment changed, however slightly. I did not follow what Madeleine Akrich (1992: 208) would call the cannula's 'script'; its inscribed or predicted way of acting in the world. Small material details meant that I was brought into a self-consciousness that made obvious what previously I had taken for granted. I was made more aware of the contours of the situation and the distance that separated me, the instrument, the patient and our environment (Ingold 2000: 414).

Both the habits developed in my environment of past practice and the ways of doing things in the environment of the moment were brought into some relief. Differences in the ward setting, how the instruments were stored and relationships with nurses and consultants were made more obvious. I felt under-qualified to be the only doctor in a hospital considering my junior status, and the discrepancies seemed to expand, gathering weight. In that moment of mismatch, I started to lose my grip not only on the tool, but also on my position in that new environment. Minute differences in equipment had led to larger effects and a series of cascading consequences.

A moment of adjustment

I started to get a little panicked. The patient needed the cannula for antibiotics that were due in half an hour and if I could not finish the job, the nurses would have to call in a doctor from the larger hospital half an hour drive away. I looked around the ward. The nurses were busy at their station. Should I ask for help? But surely this was one of my more basic jobs. I turned back to the patient, and took a deep breath.

I inspected the equipment again and practised in the air, away from the patient. I tried to get more of a feel for how the equipment moved. I decided I had room for one more attempt. I would have to go for an obvious vein that I knew would not last more than a day. The patient would have to have another cannula, but that would be tomorrow and not that evening when my blouse was soaked through with sweat and all I wanted to do was go home. I felt the patient's arm gently, looking for veins and found a large wobbly one on the back of her hand. This time the instrument moved more smoothly and blood flushed into the chamber. I slid the cannula into the vein whilst whisking out the introducer. The patient received her antibiotics, some dressings over the other punctures in her skin and an apology from me, before I burst out of the hospital into the less suffocating forest air.

During this unfortunately protracted experience for the patient, I had to adjust my technique to be able to insert the cannula. I was only able to complete the task after compromising on the positioning of the device. Rather than having someone to copy and mimic, I had to undergo my own bodily adjustment and be attentive to minute differences in sensations, the patient's body and the equipment, a subtle response and co-ordination of visual/haptic perception with action (Ingold 2000: 356).

This adjustment happened in practice. It happened through the body, as I got a measure of the instrument with my hands, incorporating myself into the new dimensions of the tool and the environment. As Ingold (2000) has discussed, skill is not a property of the individual body but rather a total system of relations, within a richly structured environment. The beginning of this chapter explored the embodiment of skills, including the use of tools, through ongoing environmentally situated practice in familiar settings. The cannulation technique I had absorbed during internship in Australia involved my hands, the instrument, a bodily memory of past patients, my ability to be able to find the equipment, my role in the hospital and a host of other environmental factors in which I dwelled. The person-tool-environment became inseparable in a familiar medical context, and fine-tuning of practice happened tacitly. The skill was learnt in an environment where it had become 'second nature', formed in, and rejuvenated in a familiar setting where all was taken for granted. In the next section I will analyse in more detail what changing contexts, what moving from one multifarious environment to another, reveals not only about these settings, but also about the nature of adjustment. I do so by drawing further upon the work of Merleau-Ponty, Ingold and Bourdieu. The chapter then extends upon that moment of mismatch, to which I argue these three theorists have given limited acknowledgement.

The atomised environment

Merleau-Ponty (1945: 160) writes that 'a movement is learned when the body has understood it, that is, when it has incorporated it into its "world"'. He suggests that to understand is to have harmony between the intention and the performance. When the body has 'ceased to be a knowing body', when it cannot draw everything together in its grip, the world becomes atomised (1945: 167, 329). He proposes that once we start to analyse an event further, the unified experience in which we are normally given over to the object, further breaks up (1945: 277).

These are some of the few instances in the *Phenomenology of Perception* in which Merleau-Ponty discusses an atomised world, being generally more interested in how one develops and retains a grip on the world, rather than loses it. Similarly, Ingold (2000: 414) only discusses losing grip briefly, in *The Perception of the Environment*, when he describes something going wrong during one of his cello performances, when he found that he became aware of himself, the instrument and the distance between them. This chapter thus extends empirically upon what has been mentioned in these theorists' work, further illuminating what happens when things become incongruent.

Bourdieu (2000) has perhaps written most substantially on what he has described as a mismatch of bodily dispositions, claiming that much of his earlier work on the *habitus* arose from such observations during fieldwork, when he was a young anthropologist in Algeria. Once again however, this term was arguably under-realised, with much empirical and theoretical work needed to flesh it out further (Noble and Watkins 2003). I suggest that by returning to Merleau-Ponty's work, which has influenced both Bourdieu's and Ingold's, that we may understand something more about adjustment during moments of mismatch. This furthers an analysis of the cannula story and our understanding of the ways in which overseas doctors adjust their embodied practice in new clinical environments.

The layered body
Merleau-Ponty (1945: 166) describes the body as having two layers, that of the habit-body, developed from past experiences, that becomes 'knowledge in the hands', and that of the body-in-the-moment. Moments of mismatch, I argue, occur when these 'layers' are incongruent, and adjustment is an oscillation between the two. Before exploring this in more detail, I will first outline what I mean by the habit-body and then by the body-in-the-moment.

The habit-body is developed in the environment that a doctor grows up and into, shaped by an intermingling and inseparable mix of wetlabs, medical schools, teachers, instruments, hospitals, the political economy of the country, disciplines studied and patients encountered. This body is developed in the richly textured environment of practice that becomes the familiar, as Merleau-Ponty (1945: 96) has put it, that 'humdrum setting which is mine'. Merleau-Ponty's notion of the habit-body became central to Bourdieu's concept of the *habitus*, in which Bourdieu (2000: 135) suggests that through sensory comprehension, the body is impressed and modified by the world around it, and thus acquires a system of dispositions attuned to the surrounding regularities. Bourdieu (2000: 138) writes that the body becomes inscribed by past experiences predisposed to react to recognised stimuli, during which the body has immediately adjusted without realising it. It is a world, Bourdieu (2000: 143) writes, that the practitioner takes for granted, because they are 'caught up in it, bound up with it; he inhabits it like a garment (*un habit*) or a familiar habitat. He feels at home in the world because the world is also in him, in the form of '*habitus*'. The habit-body and Bourdieu's extension of this, the *habitus*, helps us to understand how procedural skills become ingrained and learnt in familiar contexts.

The body-in-the-moment is similarly a practical engagement with the surrounding environment that one finds oneself in at any one time. In familiar environments, the habit-body and the body-in-the-moment are often closely aligned, leading to tacitly enacted practices. In the unfamiliar environment, the body-in-the-moment may be situated within the unexpected and one finds oneself somewhere, however slightly, 'strange'. In the moment, on that Nightingale ward, I had to get a measure of the minutely different instrument, to sense its unfamiliar tactile contours. At the same time, I had to be attentive to the patient and the texture of the environment in that cottage hospital at the edge of the oak forest.

Adjustment, I propose, is the movement between the habit-body and that body-in-the-moment, the two separated in a moment of mismatch. The cannula mismatch was made more obvious because I was an overseas doctor in an unfamiliar hospital environment. Consequently, adjustment concerns not only the present but also the past. There is an implication that immigrants cast off the baggage from their previous lives in an attempt to make a new one (Kelly and Lusis 2006: 832). Thinking about adjustment as a movement between the habit-body and the body-in-the-moment recognises that doctors come to their new workplaces with their own pasts, their own ingrained practices, and gives scope for change in practice. I have argued that adjustment reveals aspects of the overseas doctors' histories and also the new environments they find themselves in. What is revealed is not always clear – we may only get glimpses. The past is not pulled into sharp relief, nor is the present situation ever clearly delineated.

Revealing the mundane

Every practitioner in a hospital has a past repertoire of experience. Hospitals are filled with people constantly adjusting their ways of doing things, their habit-bodies with the body-in-the-moment. They are adjustments that Bourdieu (2000: 138) regards as necessities of the field. But for those in familiar contexts, this is a process that happens tacitly, in moments of minute improvisations during the evolution of skill. In the development of skilful practice we often become unconscious of the actions and processes by which we achieve the result. Polanyi (1958: 62) describes this as feeling our way to success without knowing how we do it.

It means, using the example of cannulation, that during the procedure the practitioner may respond to individual differences in patients such as co-morbid disease, previous drug use, pregnancy, age, needle-phobias and the weather, as well as other environmental conditions, all impacting on the technique used, to which practice is slightly, tacitly, tactically adjusted in response. In the *Surgeons and the Scope*, James Zetka (2003: 10) similarly details how surgeons adjust to the variable nature of the raw material of the patient's anatomy and other unexpected eventualities. He writes, 'the traits of a mature surgeon are acknowledging an obdurate, complex, and uncertain environment; adapting one's work routines to manage this environment to the best extent possible' (2003: 11). Similarly, Catherine Pope

(2002: 377–9) documents how surgical technique has to be constantly adjusted in each case, as surgeons learn to make do, drawing upon their past experiences and responses. In their study of anaesthetists, Hindmarsh and Pilnick (2007: 1413) examine the way the practitioners' bodies respond in a contingent way to moment-to-moment changes in the embodied conduct of colleagues, which they argue allows the team to seamlessly co-ordinate activities. As newcomers to a system, overseas doctors highlight these everyday practices of adjustment because of the more obvious fracture in their hospital contexts, when they are confronted with conditions quite different from those in which their *habitus* was produced (Bourdieu 2000: 161). They have to put more work into their adjusting, and thus, in the process, teach us something about it.

In the moment of mismatch the overseas doctors' series of embodied habits are interrupted, as are the normal ways of doing things in the new environment. In their adjustments, overseas doctors, like all skilled migrants, have to pay attention to how things feel, how they look, sound and smell. They have to notice 'those subtleties of texture that are all-important to good judgment and the successful practice of a craft' (Ingold 2000: 416). As Ingold writes, 'that one learns to touch, to see and to hear is obvious to any craftsman or musician . . . an "education of attention"'. Bodily adjustments in new work contexts are sensory and situated, and it is the adjustments of newcomers, in moments of mismatch, that provide us with details of this.

We can draw wider implications from this illustrative and autoethnographic study of the minutiae of medical work. Paying attention to embodied work in conditions of unfamiliarity not only teaches us about the nature of adjustment but also leaves us with important lessons about the process of situated learning. The cannulation story highlights the contextual nature of medical work, its embeddedness within a multifarious environment. There is significant social labour involved in moving medical practices from one clinical context to another, and too often this process is hidden from view in the myth of a medical universalism. Not only do skilled migrants need to be more sensitised to undertake an 'education of attention', to pay attention to details of difference that may be 'small', though large in their effect, but we also need to question our consistent attempts to standardise work practices across medical sites. Current formal assessments and regulation of overseas healthcare workers may potentially decontextualise complex processes, treating skills like pieces of luggage and ignoring the environmentally situated nature of medical practice. This can lead to serious and unfortunate clinical events.

Conclusion

Like me, few overseas doctors in the larger ethnographic study I conducted considered differences in advance. Medicine was presumed to be an abstract body of knowledge and skill that could be transported in a suitcase from place to place. But upon migration many doctors found themselves in places where patients' bodies were different, where economic resources might be more resplendent, where nurses had a different role and where there was a slightly different configuration of the cannula; aspects of the environment normally taken for granted by the 'locals' who wore it like a well-fitting white coat.

Just as objects or infrastructures become more visible during breakdowns (Star 1999: 382, Latour 2005: 81), the body becomes more visible in times of disease (Leder 1990: 87), so too do overseas doctors, moving from one context to another, reveal the taken-for-granted, seamless relations between man-tool-environment that develop through everyday practices of adjustment in hospitals. This is revealed particularly in moments of mismatch, during which the overseas doctors engage in what I have called adjustment, but which others have described as tuning (Ingold 2000), honing (Sennett 2008: 50), tinkering (Knorr-Cetina 1992) or accommodation (Pickering 1995). They are all words for describing moving between the implicit and explicit, the process of making-do, patching things together, in a moment-to-moment engagement with the environment through bodily learning and adjustment.

Whilst the contextual nature of medical practice is highlighted in this chapter, I have not argued that doctors' skills are 'context specific'. That is, I have suggested that adjustment involves a constant oscillation from a doctor's past to the present moment they find themselves in. The chapter has argued that rather than starting from scratch, skilled migrants bring with them their own ways of doing things, which they adjust in practice to meet the demands of their present situation. In this regard, they must be given more credit.

This chapter has contributed an understanding of how bodily adjustment happens in mundane medical practices, and of how procedural work is adjusted in sensory ways. How something feels, looks, sounds or smells are the important textural subtleties one needs to be attuned to when learning a craft (Ingold 2000: 416), with technology very much bound up in this process. These details are not always observable to the social scientist. They may be little changes in how things feel for the participant; small happenings that go into making adjustment dynamic. These details such as the haptic nature of fine-tuning, the perceptual registers of proprioception and pressure exerted by instruments, are the kind of sensory information that Nigel Thrift (2003) argues is missing from many accounts of practice. Exceptional studies in this area seem to lie principally in the field of music, with David Sudnow's (1978) elegant study of learning jazz improvisation through the body standing out in particular. We should be conducting more studies of this sort in medical sociology, that examine the fine grain of medical work, situating theoretically rich work within broader social and political processes.

Such future work needs to place medical practice in its embodied, sensory and environmental contexts. There is much more to develop empirically and theoretically about the ways in which embodied practices are adjusted in work settings. To do so we need to use not only methods of autoethnography, interviewing and participant observation but also incorporate creative methodologies that utilise various media such as film (Herzfeld 2009: 137), photography (Wolkowitz 2006: 33) and sound recording, which may all help to capture, however partially, the 'ineffable in mid-flight' (Herzfeld 2009: 147). Already researchers such as Erin O'Connor (2007) have used photography to illustrate the embodied learning of glass blowing, and medical sociologists have used video to help capture the 'fine-grained detail' of interactional embodied conduct in anaesthetic, surgical and ICU work settings (Iedema et al. 2006, Long et al. 2006, Hindmarsh and Pilnick 2007, Svensson et al. 2009: 890).

These methodologies raise intriguing questions regarding the nature of representation, evocation and articulation of sensory experience (Paterson 2009: 780). In exploring the possibilities of these research methods, we may need to look at how non-academics are using these methods to capture shared topics of interest (Harris 2008). For example, in relation to the photographic study of touch and the minutiae of action, Edweard Muybridge's images are an important investigation of the 'invisible' world of motion (Cresswell 2006: 61). John Berger and Jean Mohr's (1982) 'Framed portrait of a woodcutter' in *Another Way of Telling* is a wonderful exploration of *doing* work, and the way in which one's work is wrapped up in the environment that one is part of (the woodcutter's hands, the axe, chainsaw, trees and the forest). These artistic social studies flesh out embodied practices in ways which can inspire and inform our sociological enquiries.

There is much more to understand about how skills are adjusted across contexts, and how technologies become incorporated into this process. We need further studies of skilled migrants in healthcare and other work settings, which examine in detail their practices of situated learning. These studies not only need to take place in various contexts but also be constantly attentive to changing work dynamics. Institutional rearrangements, such as increased regulation and restrictions on training, are examples of ways in which the embodied nature of learning in medicine is shifting and these need to be taken into account (Nettleton *et al.* 2008). These are tasks that medical sociology has begun to embrace more fully, as evident in this collection of chapters on body work. As we further this area of research, it may be that newcomers and others on the peripheral margins of belonging, will shed much light on the minute and mundane details of healthcare practice.

Acknowledgements

I would like to thank the overseas doctors who participated in the research upon which this chapter is based. I am grateful for feedback from: Marilys Guillemin, Ali Brookes and Barbara Kamler; members of the CHS Writing Workshop, particularly Kirsten and Andrea; and finally the editors of this book and two anonymous reviewers for their insightful comments.

References

Akrich, M. (1992) The de-scription of technical objects. In Bijker, W. and Law, J. (eds) *Shaping Technology/Building Society*. Boston, Massachusetts: Institute of Technology.
Atkinson, P. (2006) Rescuing autoethnography, *Journal of Contemporary Ethnography*, 35, 4, 400–04.
Bartleet, B.-L. (2009) Behind the baton: exploring autoethnographic writing in a musical context, *Journal of Contemporary Ethnography*, 38, 6, 713–33.
Becker, H. (1970) *Sociological Work: Method and Substance*. Chicago: Aldine Publishing Company.
Berger, J. and Mohr, J. (1982) *Another Way of Telling*. New York: Pantheon.
Blaxter, M. (2009) The case of the vanishing patient? Image and experience, *Sociology of Health and Illness*, 31, 5, 762–78.
Bourdieu, P. (2000) *Pascalian Meditations*. Cambridge: Polity Press.
Conradson, D. (2003) Doing organisational space: practices of voluntary welfare in the city, *Environment and Planning A*, 35, 1975–92.
Cresswell, T. (2006) *On the Move: Mobility in the Modern Western World*, New York: Routledge.
Harris, A. (2008) The artist as surgical ethnographer: participant observers outside the social sciences, *Health: An Interdisciplinary Journal for the Social Study of Health, Illness and Medicine*, 14, 4, 501–14.
Harris, A. (2009) Overseas doctors' adjustments in Australian hospitals: an ethnographic study of how degrees of difference are negotiated in medical practice. Faculty of Medicine, University of Melbourne, PhD.
Herzfeld, M. (2009) The cultural politics of gesture: reflections on the embodiment of ethnographic practice, *Ethnography*, 10, 2, 131–52.
Hindmarsh, J. and Pilnick, A. (2007) Knowing bodies at work: embodiment and ephemeral teamwork in anaesthesia, *Organization Studies*, 28, 9, 1395–416.
Howes, D. (1995) The senses in medicine, *Culture, Medicine and Psychiatry*, 19, 125–33.

Iedema, R., Long, D. and Forsyth, R. (2006) Visibilising clinical work: video ethnography in the contemporary hospital, *Health Sociology Review*, 15, 2, 156–68.

Ingold, T. (1996) Situating action V: the history and evolution of bodily skills, *Ecological Psychology*, 8, 2, 171–82.

Ingold, T. (2000) *The Perception of the Environment: Essays on Livelihood, Dwelling and Skill*. London: Routledge.

Ingold, T. (2004) Culture on the ground: the world perceived through the feet, *Journal of Material Culture*, 9, 3, 315–40.

Kelly, P. and Lusis, T. (2006) Migration and the transnational habitus: evidence from Canada and the Philippines, *Environment and Planning A*, 38, 831–47.

Knorr-Cetina, K. (1992) The couch, the cathedral, and the laboratory: on the relationship between experiment and laboratory in science. In Pickering, A. (ed.) *Science as Practice and Culture*. Chicago: The University of Chicago Press.

Latour, B. (2005) *Reassembling the Social: an Introduction to Actor-Network-Theory*. Oxford: Oxford University Press.

Lave, J. and Wenger, E. (1994) *Situated Learning: Legitimate Peripheral Participation*. Cambridge: Cambridge University Press.

Leder, D. (1990) *The Absent Body*. Chicago: University of Chicago Press.

Long, D., Iedema, R. and Lee, B.B. (2006) Corridor conversations: clinical communication in casual spaces. In Iedema, R. (ed.) *Hospital Communication and Interaction: Professional, Managerial and Organizational Discourses and Practices in Acute Care*. Basingstoke: Palgrave Macmillan.

Merleau-Ponty, M. (1945) *Phenomenology of Perception*, New York: Routledge.

Moreira, T. (2006) Heterogeneity and coordination of blood pressure in neurosurgery, *Social Studies of Science*, 36, 1, 69–97.

Nettleton, S., Burrows, R. and Watt, I. (2008) Regulating medical bodies? The consequences of the 'modernisation' of the NHS and the disembodiment of clinical knowledge, *Sociology of Health and Illness*, 30, 3, 333–48.

Noble, G. and Watkins, M. (2003) So, how did Bourdieu learn to play tennis? Habitus, consciousness and habituation, *Cultural Studies*, 17, 3/4, 520–38.

Nutton, V. (1993) Galen at the bedside: the methods of a medical detective. In Bynum, W.F. and Porter, R. (eds) *Medicine and the Five Senses*. Cambridge: Cambridge University Press.

O'Connor, E. (2007) Embodied knowledge in glassblowing: the experience of meaning and the struggle towards proficiency, *Sociological Review*, 55, s1, 127–41.

Paterson, M. (2009) Haptic geographies: ethnography, haptic knowledges and sensuous dispositions, *Progress in Human Geography*, 33, 6, 766–88.

Pickering, A. (1995) *The Mangle of Practice: Time, Agency, and Science*. Chicago: The University of Chicago Press.

Polanyi, M. (1958) *Personal Knowledge: Towards a Post-Critical Philosophy*. London: Routledge.

Polanyi, M. (1966) *The Tacit Dimension*. London: Doubleday and Company.

Pope, C. (2002) Contigency in everyday surgical work, *Sociology of Health and Illness*, 24, 4, 369–84.

Rapport, N. (1995) Migrant selves and stereotypes: personal context in a postmodern world. In Pile, S. and Thrift, N. (eds) *Mapping the Subject: Geographies of Cultural Transformation*. New York: Routledge.

Reiser, S. (1993) Technology and the use of the senses in twentieth-century medicine. In Bynum, W.F. and Porter, R. (eds) *Medicine and the Five Senses*. Cambridge: Cambridge University Press.

Rier, D.A. (2000) The missing voice of the critically ill: a medical sociologist's first-person account, *Sociology of Health and Illness*, 22, 1, 68–93.

Sennett, R. (2008) *The Craftsman*. London: Penguin Books.

Shilling, C. (2007) Sociology and the body: classical traditions and new agendas, *Sociological Review*, 55, s1, 1–18.

Star, S.L. (1999) The ethnography of infrastructure, *American Behavioural Scientist*, 43, 3, 377–91.

Sudnow, D. (1978) *Ways of the Hand: the Organization of Improvised Conduct*. Cambridge: Harvard University Press.

Svensson, M.S., Luff, P. and Heath, C. (2009) Embedding instruction in practice: contingency and collaboration during surgical training, *Sociology of Health and Illness*, 31, 6, 889–906.

Thrift, N. (2003) Performance and . . . , *Environment and Planning A*, 35, 2019–24.

Twigg, J. (2000) Carework as a form of bodywork, *Ageing and Society*, 20, 389–411.

Williams, A. and Baláž, V. (2008) International return mobility, learning and knowledge transfer: a case of Slovak doctors, *Social Science and Medicine*, 67, 1924–33.

Wolkowitz, C. (2006) *Bodies at Work*. London: Sage Publications.

Zetka, J. (2003) *Surgeons and the Scope*. London: Cornell University Press.

11

The co-marking of aged bodies and migrant bodies: migrant workers' contribution to geriatric medicine in the UK

Parvati Raghuram, Joanna Bornat and Leroi Henry

Introduction

Adherence to an Enlightenment project which distanced itself from the uncontrollable and irrational qualities associated with the human body and, hence, an emphasis on the social, had for a long time largely excluded bodies from the sociological gaze. In the last 25 years, however, there has been a turn towards recognition of the body, especially in social theory (Turner 1984, Featherstone 1991) and feminist research (Butler 1993). Foucauldian approaches have brought the body back into social theory, by locating the body as both subject of and subjected to social and political control (Agamben 1998), while feminists have reclaimed the body as a site of struggle, emotion and representation (Grosz 1994). However, neither the Foucauldians nor the feminists pay much attention to the ageing body (Twigg 2000). It has been 'taken for granted' in health care research, 'overlooked' in community care and 'consciously ignored' in disability studies (Twigg 2002).

One exception to this is in gerontology as Twigg's (2000) and Tulle's (2008) work demonstrates. Much of this literature, however, is marked by tensions between the biological and social determinants of how the ageing body is constituted, so that it rarely becomes anything other than a site of either unfettered agency or abjectness. In this chapter we explore the experiences of geriatricians who recuperated ageing bodies from abjectness to agency through their medical practices. While geriatricians have to deal with ageing bodies which are impaired and disabled, it is through the healing work they do on such bodies, that the careers of geriatricians are defined and success valued. As in other sectors of body work, working out a better body is part of, and essential to, geriatric practice. Yet, the limits of an ageing body and the stigma that subsequently attaches to older bodies, means that geriatric medicine came to be populated by bodies that were themselves marked, even stigmatised – the racialised bodies of South Asians (Ministry of Health 1976, Smith 1980, Rivett 1998). This chapter explores what happened when racialised bodies and older bodies, both of which are often seen as marginalised, came into relation with each other in the second half of the 20th century. We suggest that rather than a double marginalisation, these two marked bodies were both recuperated through this association. In this chapter we use the word recuperation to mean both the physical restoration of some bodies but also the ways

Body Work in Health and Social Care, First Edition. Edited by Julia Twigg, Carol Wolkowitz, Rachel Lara Cohen and Sarah Nettleton.

in which the meanings of both the black and ageing bodies were improved through this restoration. It involved a reconfiguration of the status of both sets of bodies.

The chapter draws on two sets of oral history interviews: with doctors who pioneered the development of geriatric medicine in the UK in the 1950s to 1970s; and with South Asian overseas-trained doctors who later peopled the profession, especially between the mid-1960s and mid-1980s. These doctors, who had themselves experienced distance and discrimination, look back at their careers to provide evidence of how they contributed to the emergence and development of geriatric medicine, a specialty marked by stigma and marginalisation. This allows us to see how the medical care of older people is very much an embodied experience for both doctors and patients. We seek an understanding of geriatric medicine as a site where the identities of the two marked bodies are interlinked but are also rescripted through the 'figure' of the recuperable aged body. We also draw on archival sources which illustrate debate and discussion amongst policy makers and members of the medical profession contemporary to the interview evidence.

We begin with a brief overview of social gerontology's engagement with the body in late life, then go on to consider the racialised bodies of those engaged in their care, to briefly introduce how these two literatures have dealt with the body. These literatures suggest that although the body is a rich site of theorising, bringing the two together can advance existing analysis of the points at which the two bodies meet. In particular, it can offer a way of extending the possibilities of biological understandings of advanced ageing and contributions made by geriatricians to this field through insights from new theories of race and the notion of assemblage therein (Deleuze and Guattari 1987). This juxtaposition of the two literatures offers us a way of moving beyond a theorisation of these bodies primarily as sites of marginalisation. In the following sections this argument is illustrated through the use of examples from the two datasets. Thinking of the body as an assemblage with many elements, some of which are stigmatised but which can nevertheless be recuperated, helps us to think beyond stigma in the context of body work and to see how the meanings of these bodies are rearranged in social space. The chapter thus contributes to current theorisation of embodiment by offering an example of new ways of rethinking the link between black and ageing bodies.

Ageing and the body in social gerontology

Gerontologists have vastly contributed to understandings of attitudes to the ageing body. However, engagements with the biological and medical aspects of physical change in late life tend not to be included by either of the two main perspectives adopted: political economist and postmodern views. On the one hand, early materialist explanations rooted in a political economy position saw old age and older people as marginalised and disempowered by social class, labour market exclusion and welfare policies, resulting in a structured dependency (Phillipson and Walker 1986). In contrast, social constructionist (postmodern) theorists position age as a set of socially constructed discursive practices that are determined by and determining of older people. Criticising materialist arguments for the ways in which old age is seen as structurally limiting, postmodern theorising in gerontology highlights ways in which older people are actively engaged in choosing their life styles through a 'Third Age' with its own patterns of consumption, finding ways to escape or opt out of the imposition of culturally determined age stages and signs of ageing (Gilleard 2002, Estes *et al.* 2003: 90). Both, however, in their different ways, render the body invisible, effectively distancing from view a Fourth Age of dependency and impairment (Higgs and Jones 2008: 75–6).

As Twigg has argued, political economy arguments adopted by some social gerontologists, focus on the structural inhibitions which dominate such bodies. They have almost given in to an ageism, which sees the older body as marked in a negative way, thus, contributing to a further downgrading of older people (Twigg 2004: 60). The body has come to be seen as a passive receptor of age, sometimes alongside class, gender and disability. Even though some of those who earlier espoused a political economy of old age, have shifted their ground to embrace what they describe as a critical gerontological perspective, uniting political economy with biographical approaches, and arguments which focus on social, historical and cultural change (Phillipson and Biggs 1998: 12, Phillipson 2008), the body still remains out of engagement. Though arguing that social constructionism approaches risk '. . . ignoring both structural inequalities and the threats to identity posed by an uncertain social environment' (Phillipson and Biggs 1998: 20), the bodily experience of ageing is not presented as a contributory factor, even when informed by biography. Indeed, evidence from research drawing on life histories and diary-based data suggests that biographically based accounts tend to disembody lives into longer-term temporal framings, with practical and somatic aspects of ageing playing only indicative roles (Bornat and Bytheway 2010).

Postmodern arguments which engage with such practices as the reversioning of a life through consumption patterns, also have their limits. They are less able to explain biologically determined events relating to the body such as a fall. Similarly, the notion of a confected 'mask' of youth, can lead to the concealing of an older identity. It runs the risk of creating a set of signs and cultural references which exclude old age and ageing, leaving an empty space where an older self might be (Biggs 2004: 49, Gilleard and Higgs 2007).

Where the gerontologists of all persuasions find common ground is in discussions of medical interventions which seek to hold back, eliminate or compensate for the effects of ageing. As Vincent (2008) highlights, such attempts to control biological ageing, or 'biogerontology', are deeply imbued with ageist attitudes and are part of an anti-ageing culture that generates fears, prejudice and anxiety about growing old, especially those signs of ageing which signal a fourth age of frailty and impairment. Vincent (2007) goes on to argue for de-coupling science from an ageist culture by revaluing the processes of life and death and accepting their interdependence.

A critique of a determinist link between science and ageing can also be seen in social gerontology. So, for example, Estes and Binney (1989), in their discussion of the 'biomedical paradigm', suggest that the 'science of ageing' operates as '. . . a dominant and powerful mode of thought in Western industrialised societies . . .' with the result that old age is defined as 'a process of basic, inevitable, relatively immutable biological phenomena' (1989: 588). On her part, Twigg combines opposition to medicalisation with a patriarchal analysis, castigating 'traditional gerontology' for neglecting the body and thus 'effectively handing the topic to medicine, which is staffed by high-status male doctors' (2004: 68). Others, such as Gilleard and Higgs (2007) go further, arguing that the care practices of geriatricians have resulted in the continued institutionalisation of older people in settings where they are segregated and where, as a result of physical and mental impairment, they are observed and assessed. They suggest that 'If reflexivity is the marker of modernity, empowering the agency of the third age, the fourth age is marked by its negation' (2007: 17).

The gerontologist Stephen Katz (1996) is unusual for his linking of gerontology and geriatric medicine. Arguing that these two disciplines, one social, the other medical, complement each other historically and theoretically, he shows how each has an interest in identifications and categorisation, both emerging as discrete disciplines at around the same time in the 20th century. The geriatric medicine that Katz describes emerged in the UK as a system of classification which sought ways to deal with frail older bodies, secluded, as we shall see, within settings offering only basic care. Marjory Warren, who pioneered this approach in the UK in the late 1930s, observing patients on wards which she, as a doctor, had been allocated, divided patients up into five groups: 'Chronic up-patients'; 'Chronic continent bed-ridden patients'; 'Chronic incontinent patients'; 'Senile, quietly restless and mentally confused or childish patients' and 'Senile dements'. Her assessment, based on this classification, led to a 25 per cent discharge rate as patients were presented with rehabilitation programmes and activity instead of bed rest (Warren 1942: 822, Barton and Mulley 2003). Building on her work, other geriatricians, as Katz argues, developed a medicine which depended on the identification of 'the aged body' as 'a system of signification' (with particular and recognisable features), as 'separate' (requiring its own treatments and associated practices) and as 'dying' (identifying the effects of degeneration and the inevitability of death as part of life) (1996: 40–41). Katz' positioning of geriatric medicine within a broader medical and social landscape is helpful in highlighting how to move beyond the inabilities of both materialist and postmodern approaches to take into account and theorise the impaired ageing body. It opens up the body to multiple forms of signification but does not take it further. Moreover, what is still lacking in his and other theorising is an understanding of geriatric medicine as more than a set of practices. In such a way, without its practitioners, it too is disembodied.

Migration, race and the body

Like gerontology, migration research has become increasingly interested in the body (*e.g.* see chapters from this book). One reason for interest in migration and the body is the recognition of the embodied nature of work that migrants often perform. The extraction of bodily labour has always been part of capitalist exploitation but in a globalising world, the fields of exploitation have expanded and incorporated migrants in new ways (Wolkowitz 2006). One field where migrants undertake this body work is in the care of older people. An increase in the numbers of older people who require help and support concomitant with a proportionate decrease in those available or willing to take on such work, paid or unpaid (Bond and Cabrero 2007: ch 6), has meant that this 'undesirable' work is increasingly being done by migrants in the UK (Doyle and Timonen 2009). Changing demographic patterns such as an increase in the older population as well as a decrease in the number of women who can provide care for such people, because of both geographical mobility and the increasing numbers of women employed in paid work, has meant that the nexus between migration, care and the body has become an important area of research in health and social policy, feminist research, and in migration studies. One finding of this research is that the work being done by migrants, especially migrant women, is dirty, dangerous and difficult (Anderson 2000).

Interestingly, the body has also returned to the theoretical fold of race in new ways. Through the early part of the 20th century, race was theorised as biological difference. Descriptions of behaviour and dispositions were posited on racialised bodies. For instance, blackness was tied in essentialist ways to activities such as crime as if they were innate traits of black bodies. In response, through the 1970s and 1980s a social constructionist, anti-essentialist model of race was fostered both within race theory and in anti-racist politics in order to counter this version of race. It aimed to take the 'problem of race' away from racialised bodies alone to think about how race was discursively constituted, especially in representational practices. As such, and drawing on poststructuralist theory, the complexities of blackness were identified as much and through the politics of whiteness. The problems lay in the ways in which black bodies were being scripted as associated with negative values. As Yancy (2008) argues 'whiteness comes replete with its assumptions for what to expect of a Black body (or non-white body), how dangerous and unruly it is, how unlawful, criminal and hypersexual it is. The discourse and comportment of whites are shaped through tacit racist scripts, calcified modes of being, that enable them to sustain and perpetuate their whitely-being-in-the-world' (2008: 846). However, as Pitcher (2009) has argued, these theorisations were embedded in their own materialities – of what was necessary at the time in order to unsettle existing ways of appropriating the black body.

But times have changed. More recently, a certain kind of anti-racism has become hegemonic, with its mantras widely repeated and appropriated without changing racist practices. The way in which 'construction' was analysed in social constructionist theories opened up possibilities of incorporation of what was an essentially anti-racist theory by closet racists (Pitcher 2009), suggesting the need to return to recognising the 'ways in which the materiality of bodies matter to the production of racial categories and meanings' (Veninga 2008: 108). Towards this, race theorists argue that race is not simply linguistically constructed or socially organised but is a bodily event, that is shaped by the phenomenology of the phenotype (Saldanha 2006). Phenotype is thus once again important in analysing race although it involves new ways of theorising the body. However, as Saldanha argues this understanding of race must be reontologised, 'The concept of race is not for taxonomic ordering, but for studying the *movements between* [his emphasis] human bodies, things, and their changing environment' (Saldanha 2006: 11). Some of this new theorisation of race has drawn on Judith Butler's theories of performativity to show how racialised identities are lived out through a set of embodied practices (Veninga 2008). Others have drawn on phenomenology to recognise the ways in which even knowledge of the discursive nature of race does not inhibit bodily responses of rejection and fear from white bodies (Yancy 2008, Ahmed 2007). It takes us back, albeit in new ways, to the body that Fanon evokes in *Black Skin, White Masks* (1986). However, now it is not only the black body that is made conscious of its existence but rather an attempt is made to force open for interrogation the habituations of white bodies' responses to black skin.

This white response is also theorised as the response to seeing the black body's presence as an incursion, as out of place (Puwar 2004). Ahmed (2007) outlines how 'stop and search' is a way of apprehending this dislocated body, but also how this process of stopping, is a way of hailing, of recruiting into this place the black body that is stopped and searched. It disorientates the black body and is remembered because it has both a physical and an affective register. It is expressed, enacted but also recalled. The white response has effects on the black body. However, as Saldanha (2006) argues, both the white response and the black body are not fixed but rather a 'chain of contingency' (2006: 18). Saldanha draws on Deleuze and Guattari's (1987) notion of machinic assemblage to argue that race is a heterogeneous assemblage of aspects like DNA, phenotype, political and cultural practices and discursive framings that come together in ways that are influenced by their common, repeated attractions. There is a viscosity to these practices so that they frequently appear in similar constellations. Hence, white or pale skin is often tied together with other elements of the racial assemblage. But not always. The assemblage also has emergent properties, its elements come together in new ways in different circumstances.

One site where these elements come together is in the care of old people. In migrant carework these two forms of bodies, both out of place, are brought together. Migrant bodies are often (but not always) somatically marked and, in the case we describe below, racialised as 'brown', 'coloured', 'black' or othered in some visible way.[1] Moreover, for many migrants the work they do, caring for those who are most dependent, including body work of touching and cleaning dirty or frail bodies, means that they too bear the negative ascriptions of their work (Dyer *et al.* 2008). Working in sites that are sometimes considered 'out of place' such as hospitals and care settings intensified this demeaning positioning. Both black bodies and older bodies are marked by disgust and a distancing from the desirable body. This may be due to phenotypical variation as in race or to the effects of change and impairment as in the ageing body. Thus, both bodies, singly and in association, are seen as out of place, never ordinary and always questioned and classified in some way. This set of characteristics seems to come together (with viscosity, as Saldanha would argue) to dominate a particular way of thinking about both black and old bodies. A particular assemblage appears to dominate both types of bodies in a stigmatising way.

In this chapter, however, we want to look at how we can unsettle these bodily understandings through rescripting the bodily presence of migrants through the saga of the recuperable body of older ill people. The emergent elements of the assemblage that makes up both the older body and the black body are, at least in part, rewritten. Here, associations with particular groups of cared-for people and situations where care is produced and reproduced have outcomes, both for the bodies of migrants and those for whom they care. Towards this we revisit the history of the geriatric specialty through the experiences of those who successively worked on its development.

The project

The chapter draws on secondary analysis of interviews conducted by Margot Jefferys with the pioneers of geriatric medicine in the UK and with a new dataset of interviews with South Asian geriatricians, who played a central part in its development.[2] The first dataset comprises 72 interviews which Professor Margot Jefferys and colleagues carried out in 1990–91 with the founders of the geriatric specialty. Between them they cover the history of developments in the health care of older people from the late 1930s to the end of the 1980s. This was a period of profound change in health policy in the UK. The interviews reveal attitudes and practice in the care of one of the most marginal of all patient groups, frail older people.

The Jefferys interviews with pioneers included only one doctor of South Asian origin. The second dataset addresses this deficiency by generating oral history interviews between 2007 and 2009 with 60 retired and serving South Asian geriatricians.[3] Interviewees for this second project were recruited through networks of overseas doctors (British Association of Physicians of Indian Origin for example), the British Geriatrics Society and through snowballing as the project progressed. Both interview schedules used a life-history approach, asking participants to talk about their childhood, upbringing, education at school and college and subsequent training and careers. In the case of the South Asian doctors they were also asked about their training in their home countries and after arrival in the UK and about their reasons for migration to the UK, arrival and subsequent career progression in the UK with a focus on opportunities, barriers and sources of support (for a discussion of our use of the two datasets see Bornat forthcoming).

Our interviewees included doctors trained in India, Bangladesh, Sri Lanka, Pakistan and Burma, ranging in age between 40 and 91 and arriving in the UK from the early 1950s onwards. Two-thirds of the interviewees were retired, semi-retired or arrived in the UK prior to 1976. All except one had worked as consultants and some also held academic posts such as that of professors. All except five of the interviewees were male.[4] The interviewees were geographically dispersed but with clusters in the North West, Wales and the northern fringes of London. The interviews reflect on the ways in which networks operated to influence labour market outcomes through the second half of the 20th century.

These sources have been supplemented by documentary evidence from the archives of the British Geriatric Society, British Medical Association, Institute of Commonwealth Studies and relevant Ministry of Health, Foreign Office and other records housed at the National Records Office. Together they provide official narratives of the contexts within which migration, geriatric medicine (particularly staffing levels and resources) and thus the bodies of practitioners and patients were being discussed during the second half of the 20th century.

Geriatric medicine and the older body

Interviews with the pioneers of geriatric medicine provide us with dramatic accounts of the impact of their first encounters with the medical care of chronically sick older people. They reinforce Katz's (1996) arguments about the importance of characterisation and spatial separation of different kinds of ageing bodies. However, Katz' analysis does not allow for personal experience, the subjectivity of the doctors and their observations and perspectives. Samuel Vine, interviewed for the Jefferys study, recounts an early experience and personal turning point, when, as a newly qualified doctor, Cambridge educated and having served with the British Army in the Far East during World War Two, he secured a medical registrarship at Fulham Hospital in London in the early years of the NHS. His consultant explained an aspect of his job:

'Oh look, there's one frightful little chore that you have to do. I'm awfully sorry but somewhere', he said 'I've never been in them, of course, but somewhere in, in this hospital, in the Fulham Hospital, there are what are called the chronic sick wards'.

And he said 'Look, all you've got to do is find an hour or so on an alternate Thursday afternoon, just pop in there, have a word with the sister, see if there's anything she wants, it's mainly repeating prescriptions, I think that's all you have to do. . . .

And I had a look in and I went back, I think possibly visibly shaken, to the charming Irish sister, red-headed Irish sister . . . and she said 'Would you like a cup of tea?' I said 'yes please'.

And so she said 'Now I've got these prescription forms for you to sign', and, do you know, I was just about to do it and I said 'Wait a minute, sister, I have never in my life yet signed a prescription for a patient whom I have not seen and I'm not going to start this afternoon. I will see all these patients before I sign these prescriptions'.

And the sister nearly fainted at that point because this was the first time any doctor had insisted on seeing the patients.

Well, I was shocked, amazed, appalled, saddened and very upset at what I saw that afternoon. I could not believe that within the campus of one hospital, two separate standards should exist for treatment based solely upon age, 65 for men and '60 for women'.

(Dr Samuel Vine, b 1919, qualified 1943, consultant, main career Oxford, interviewed by Anthea Holme 17.05.1991, Oral History of Geriatrics as a Medical Specialty, Jefferys collection, British Library C512/68/01-02).

This encounter with the ageing body and the conditions and contexts of its existence were, for many of the early geriatricians, the turning point that led to involvement and leadership in the development of the discipline. They had to argue for moving geriatrics away from simply signing prescriptions to active engagement with the bodily impairment including seeing and diagnostic touching. Their aim, as some argue, was to develop a more humane and egalitarian access to healthcare suited to the needs of older bodies (Thane 2000, Barton and Mulley 2003). However, other historians argue that the main motivation, sometimes understated sometimes openly articulated, was the removal of older people from hospital beds, dealing with 'bed blocking', thought to be the main obstacle to more effective resource management in the emergent health service (Hall and Bytheway 1982, Barker 1987, Bridgen 2001).

Separation and marking out of older bodies was, as argued by Katz, central to the development of the discipline, although as Dr Ferguson Anderson (the first professor of elderly medicine appointed in Scotland in 1965) interviewed by Jefferys, reflecting on Warren's classification of chronically sick older bodies suggests, there was an imperative behind this categorisation. The aim was to find out who might be rehabilitated and who required long-term care, and to make a case for the recuperation of the older body, medically and in terms of simple justice, as shown below:

> . . . the only way to protect the elderly was to give them special entry to a unit so they didn't stand in line with the young, because if they stood in line with the young they would never get in. And that was human justice.

> But the elderly deserved a bit of justice too.

> (Professor Sir Ferguson Anderson, b 1913, qualified 1936, consultant, main career Glasgow, interviewed by Margot Jefferys 19.04.1991, Jefferys collection, British Library C512/23/01)

Nineteen-forty seven saw the establishment of the first organisation of doctors specialising in the care of older people, The Medical Society for the Care of the Elderly (later the British Geriatrics Society), and over the following 20 years, initiatives and practices developed that marked older bodies as different and categorisable. These included age-related admissions procedures, separate provision within geriatric units, day hospitals for older people living in the community and rehabilitation facilities introduced and managed by a growing number of consultant geriatricians.

Geriatric medicine developed in relation to bodies with specific and observable characteristics (Katz 1996). Ferguson Anderson explains how this meant knowing the ageing body in such a way that:

> . . . the doctor in geriatric medicine may know more about incontinence or mental confusion than . . . the person working only with younger people.

> And so it was two-fold: it was to get beds put aside for the waiting lists which occurred and it was the accumulation of knowledge and team work that began to make us feel that we could hold our heads up and that we were better at it.

> (Ferguson Anderson)

This was knowledge that recognised the finitude and the temporal limits to the body (Katz 1996) but also its possibilities. John Fry, one of the Jefferys' interviewees, takes a position that echoes a continuing controversy relating to intervention:

And I think the other common sense situation is that one has to accept that one is dealing with a body that's ageing. . . . I find I have an important role now as a protector of my patients from over-enthusiastic cardiologists who think that they ought to put everyone on treadmills and angiograms and operations and angioplasts, rather than to try and be more commonsensical and manage the disease as it occurs in a person of that particular age . . .

(Dr John Fry, b 1922, qualified 1944, general practitioner, main career Croydon, interviewed by Margot Jefferys 17.04.1991, Jefferys collection, British Library C512/23/01)

Geriatricians thus advocated what is special, separate and appropriate for the aged body. So much for the origins and development of the geriatric specialty, but how was it peopled and what were the conditions under which it was practised?

Geriatric medicine and racialised migrant bodies

Promoting the specialty as having a particular knowledge and set of skills and with a campaigning and advocating edge that set it very distinctively against other medical specialties was not enough to make it attractive to new medical graduates in the early years. Recruitment was to be problematic. The very marginal nature of frail bodies in the medical system, the disregard they experienced and the assumptions as to the kind of medicine that might be practised all conspired to negatively mark the specialty and, with the exception of some who attained eminence more generally, those doctors who practised it. The body of the geriatrician was thus from the start marked and influenced by and through its relation with the ageing body. Thus, Vine relates this encounter with his consultant at the start of his medical career in the early 1950s, which was typical of attitudes expressed:

. . . he said 'We haven't really discussed what you're going to do with your medical future, I've never known whether to advise you to be a cardiologist or a gastroenterologist'. And I said 'Well I think I'm going to probably be a little bit of everything, because, although the term general physician is now gradually becoming a little bit of a misnomer, there is need for physicians for the care of the elderly, and I think that I want to spend my time as a physician in geriatric medicine'.

He said 'Oh', he said, 'what a waste', I said 'Oh no it is not'. I said 'Look, I've seen so much that I must at least get this out of my system now'.

(Samuel Vine)

Thus, in constructing this discipline, the characteristics of the ageing body also diffused to mark those who cared for them.[5] Typically, interviewees found that it was a low-status specialty and it therefore came to be populated by people who for various reasons had found they had little scope for career progression in a preferred medical specialty. Some had been demobbed late at the end of World War Two, others were refugees, some had worked abroad, although others had decided to specialise in a new and growing specialty after encountering an earlier pioneer and whose methods were more inspiring than those of the general consultant physicians they had worked with. Geriatric medicine was both a site of stigma and of opportunity for advancement for these doctors.

Geriatric medicine, however, operated in similar ways for other doctors who also found it difficult to make their way in the health service – racialised, migrant doctors, who found their career paths blocked in other disciplines:

Now in 74/75/76 if you applied for – there were popular jobs – if you applied for obstetrics, gynaecology being an Indian you hardly ever got it. If you did you got it and you stayed at SHO level, you didn't get a Registrar job. And to get a Registrar job would have been extremely difficult. There were, there were instances where the Consultants said 'I have shortlisted, this is my shortlist. I have included all those that I could – the names I could pronounce and spell'.

(Dr Dwarak Sastry, b 1945 India, arrived in UK 1973, consultant physician in geriatrics, main career Cardiff, interviewed by Leroi Henry 21.01.2008, British Library Overseas trained South Asian Geriatricians interview, SAG collection, British Library C512/08/01-02)

The people 'whose names they could not pronounce or spell' therefore congregated in the less desirable specialties such as geriatric medicine where staffing was an issue.

As John Agate, interviewed for the Jefferys project, suggested:

Well, yes. One of the problems has been that staffing of geriatric departments hasn't always been easy, we have had to appoint quite a lot of doctors from the Indian sub-continent to be registrars and even senior registrars, so for quite a period the only applicants for consultant jobs were in fact not British citizens trained by British methods.

They had been to respectable geriatric departments and learnt the trade but when they got appointed to x, y, z, they had Indian or Pakistani names or whatever else. And it tended to get known as the sort of, you know, dark-skinned specialty.

(Dr John Agate, b 1919, qualified c.1943, consultant, main career Ipswich, interviewed by Hazel Houghton 03.05.1991, Jefferys collection, British Library C512/08/01-02)

There are many similar stories narrated by the South Asian geriatricians interviewed for our project, but if we stay with these accounts we only reverberate the familiar stories of marked aged and racialised bodies. Our interest lies in taking things further to suggest that despite the extent to which there is a double marginalisation implied in this relationship between black and ageing bodies, thinking of these bodies as an assemblage, also presented opportunities for a remixing of the elements that make up these bodies. They could come together in new and different forms of association.

On the one hand, the association between racialised bodies and older bodies provoked concern for the welfare of older bodies as noted in the minutes of this meeting between senior officers at the Department of Health and Social Security (DHSS) and Regional Medical Officers. They record a Dr Whittaker's concern that:

. . . 55 per cent of senior registrarships and 85 per cent of registrarships were occupied by overseas graduates (therefore) it was apparent that Geriatric medicine was in imminent danger of becoming an 'overseas' specialty. Such a state of affairs was in his opinion unfair and unacceptable to the senior citizens of our society'.

(DHSS 1975: 4)

Here we see the joining together of two irredeemable bodies being presented as problematic, but with the separation of the two being proposed as salvation for the 'senior citizen'.

The South Asian doctors, however, also recognised the potential that lay in this story of salvation and decided to find career progression through it. They were acutely aware of how older bodies were received and treated in the NHS and used it as a site of possibilities. For instance, when a male South Asian geriatrician (now aged 82) encountered geriatric medicine, he also decided what *he* wanted from it:

> So anyway he (his consultant) sent me down to then see Ferguson Anderson . . . And he was good. And I learned a bit. . . . And . . . my boss said '[nickname], the coming up specialty is geriatrics. It is now opening its doors. Money will flood if you are good. But that is something you could do' . . . I saw Ferguson Anderson's unit. Lots of elderly people. Some degree of medicine and majority looking after them, which I didn't want to do.
>
> (Dr L028, b 1927 India, arrived in UK 1953, retired consultant geriatrician, main career North West of England, interviewed by Leroi Henry 22.04.2008, SAG collection, British Library C1356/12)[6].

This South Asian geriatrician then went on to talk about how there was a post in old Egypt known as 'a keeper of the bones'. When pharaohs died young, these keepers were buried with them but this geriatrician did not want to be 'keeper of the bones'. He wanted to mend them if he could because that is what he fought for, qualified for!

Opportunities for personal and professional development were, in the South Asian interviews, often linked with accounts of how perceptions of and the commitment to those aged bodies was more than simply a way up the ladder of the medical hierarchy. It was also a search for more egalitarian and effective ways of working with older bodies, to change the status quo, as evidenced below. In this lengthy extract, one of us speaks to a male South Asian geriatrician who first came to the UK in 1967, who reminisces about a patient whom he treated in the early 1970s:

> So I got the first patient, not just back, it took me five years but I got him back to work . . . I'm not joking, I cried that day. I cried that day when that fellow – he was a butcher – I got him back to work . . . I will never forget what he told me, he was a cantankerous man, he was extremely antagonistic to medical profession, he felt medical profession let him down you see. Single man, hard drinking, hard working . . . And I always examined every patient I ever transferred from anybody else. Very detailed examination. He would not allow me to examine him. I'll never forget his words. Do you know what he told me? 'What can you fucking black bastard do for me?' That was his approach to me. Exact words I am repeating. Do you know, I liked what he said. This man was a fighting spirit. And I was looking for a guy I can work on who has spirits and he was the first person to express it. I said 'I am going to pick on this guy'. It took me about a month before he allowed me to touch him. I am not joking. I used to go 'Good morning' he used to turn away. Eventually I said 'Good morning' and he said it back and I said 'Look, let me have a look at you' . . . I used to go and chat with him, sit with him and talk to him, and he knew he was getting better. He worked like mad. Gradually the power returned. Never came back to full but he could walk with two sticks in the end.

(Dr. A.K. Viswan, b 1941 India, arrived UK 1968, consultant physician, main career West Midlands, interviewed by Parvati Raghuram 18.11.08, SAG collection, British Library C1356/13)

The geriatricians worked with bodies, largely through diagnostic touching, using such touch to understand the bodies and to work out forms of treatment. They used their understanding of how bodies work to identify what kinds of work should be done to make the older body work better. And it was through this that the geriatrician gained recognition and a sense of personal achievement.

The pioneers of geriatric medicine and the first wave of overseas-trained South Asian doctors might applaud the range and types of healthcare provision for older people in the first years of the 21st century, feeling themselves vindicated in their push for fairer and better treatment and care. However, they might also be alarmed to see and hear that there is still some way to go before equal access to good and sensitively delivered healthcare is available to frail older patients. Ageism dies hard, as reports of scandals, inhumane treatment and struggles over resources in accounts from relatives, care workers, geriatricians and older people make clear (McVeigh 2002, House of Commons 2007, Skellington 2008, National Pensioners Convention 2009). Racism too continues to mar the health service. Under these conditions it might be said that recuperation of both bodies has been partial, with continuing implications for frail patients as well as for racialised migrant doctors.

Conclusion

In this chapter we draw on an ESRC-funded research project and the data therein to juxtapose the experiences of older bodies and the racialised migrant bodies who cared about them. We argue that through the encounter between these bodies, the older body came to be increasingly seen as a body that could be cured and recuperated, while this process of recuperation also gave geriatricians a distinctive place and recognition in the medical specialty. Thus, the two bodies, which are usually seen in negative ways, came together in meaningful ways. Geriatricians have, through their work, shifted the position of the 'event horizon' that separates off a Fourth Age (Higgs and Jones 2008: 105) and have thus intervened in the mutual reinforcement of the marking that accompanied ageing, and hence the careers of those who cared for such ageing bodies.

Phenotypical variations and age variations are both caught up in competition for resources. It is a willingness to look for bodily recuperations that has interested us. Drawing on data from the two sets of interviews, we argue the need to consider the agentic ways in which a group of migrant doctors took advantage of disadvantage to contribute to practices which resulted in changes in the way the aged body was and is recognised. The racialised body works on an ageing body and both are recuperated in this encounter, through the connections they make, pointing to the need to go beyond the obvious significations of race and age, and suggesting that bodies can connect in new and unexpected ways. Bodies do not necessarily contain the possibilities for who you are – these possibilities are made. By thinking of the bodies that are involved in body work as assemblages of different elements, the negativity that is associated with ageing and racialised bodies is given room for reconfiguration and recuperation. This reading is a way of thinking beyond the necessary association between stigma, age and race. It is a step towards seeing the many different ways in which the connections between differently marked bodies could be made and towards proliferating our thinking of body work.

Acknowledgements

We would like to acknowledge the support of the ESRC in funding this research (ESRC grant reference number: RES-062-23-0514), and Margot Jefferys, her colleagues and the British Library for access to the dataset on the pioneers of geriatrics. We would also like to thank all the interviewees who have participated in the two projects.

Notes

1   As Datta and Brickell (2008) demonstrate, issues of racialisation also exist for the large numbers of Eastern European migrants who have migrated since 2004 to work in the UK. However, this chapter does not deal with the issue of European whiteness and how this is negotiated in relation to the racial superiority of Englishness.
2   The Jefferys collection is deposited at the British Library as 'Oral History of Geriatrics as a Medical Specialty' (collection ref. C512). The South Asian Geriatricians collection is also deposited at the British Library as 'Overseas trained South Asian Geriatricians interviews' (collection ref. C1356).
3   'Overseas-trained South Asian doctors and the development of geriatric medicine', ESRC grant reference number: RES-062-23-0514.
4   Feminists have made important contributions to theorising bodies but in this chapter we have focused on the intersection between age and race, and not included gender. The extracts used in the chapter were, however, all from men.
5   The reduced opportunities to do private practice and the poor physical environments where geriatric medicine was practised also influenced the status of geriatrics.
6   Some of the South Asian interviewees requested anonymity for their interview and recording.

References

Agamben, G. (1998) *Homo Sacer: Sovereign Power and Bare Life*. Stanford: Stanford University Press.
Ahmed, S. (2007) A phenomenology of whiteness, *Feminist Theory*, 8, 149–68.
Anderson, B. (2000) *Doing the Dirty Work? The Global Politics of Domestic Labour*. London: Zed Books.
Barker, W.H. (1987) *Adding Life to Years: Organised Geriatric Services in Great Britain and Implications for the United States*. Baltimore: The Johns Hopkins University Press.
Barton, A. and Mulley, G. (2003) History of the development of geriatric medicine in the UK, *Postgraduate Medical Journal*, 79, 229–34.
Biggs, S. (2004) Age, gender, narratives, and masquerades, *Journal of Aging Studies*, 18, 45–58.
Bond, J. and Cabrero, G.R. (2007) Health and dependency in later life. In Bond, J., Peace, S., Dittman-Kohli, F. and Westerhof, G. (eds) *Ageing in Society*. London: Sage.
Bornat, J. (forthcoming) Revisiting the archives – opportunities and challenges: a case study from the history of geriatric medicine, in *Secondary Analysis*, Centre for Ageing and Biographical Studies and Centre for Policy on Ageing, publication 12 in the series The Representation of Older People in Ageing Research.
Bornat, J. and Bytheway, B. (2010) Perceptions and presentations of living with everyday risk in later life, British Journal of Social Work Advance Access published on January 27, 2010. doi:10.1093/bjsw/bcq001.
Bridgen, P. (2001) Hospitals, geriatric medicine, and the long-term care of elderly people, *Social History of Medicine*, 14, 3, 507–52.
British Geriatrics Society (1975) Working party on geriatric medicine, aspects of recruitment and relationship to general medicine, File I 12/228, British Geriatrics Society archives.

Butler, J. (1993) *Bodies that Matter*. New York: Routledge.
Datta, A. and Brickell, K. (2008) 'We have a little bit more finesse, as a nation': constructing the Polish worker on London's building sites, *Antipode*, 41, 3, 439–464.
Deleuze, G. and Guattari, F. (1987) *A Thousand Plateaus: Capitalism and Schizophrenia*. Minneapolis: University of Minnesota Press.
Denham, M.J. (2004) The history of geriatric medicine and hospital care of the elderly in England between 1929 and the 1970s. Unpublished PhD thesis, University College, London.
Department of Health and Social Security (1975) Medical manpower policy in relation to the National Health Service, Notes of a meeting, File I 12/224. British Geriatrics Society archives.
Doyle, M. and Timonen, V. (2009) The different faces of care work: understanding the experiences of the multi-cultural care workforce, *Ageing and Society*, 29, 3, 337–50.
Dyer, S., McDowell, L. and Batnitzky, A. (2008) Emotional labour/body work: the caring labours of migrants in the UK's National Health Service, *Geoforum*, 39, 6, 2030–8.
Estes, C. and Binney, E. (1989) The biomedicalization of aging: dangers and dilemmas, *The Gerontologist*, 29, 5, 587–96.
Estes, C., Biggs, S. and Phillipson, C. (2003) *Social Theory, Social Policy and Ageing: a critical introduction*. Maidenhead: Open University Press.
Fanon, F. (1986) *Black Skin, White Masks*. London: Pluto Press.
Gilleard, C. (1996) Consumption and identity in late life: toward a cultural gerontology, *Ageing and Society*, 16, 4, 489–98.
Gilleard, C. and Higgs, P. (1996) Geriatrics: the rise and fall of medicine for old age? Paper presented at the Annual Conference of the British Society of Gerontology, Manchester.
Gilleard, C. and Higgs, P. (2007) Ageing without agency: theorizing the fourth age'. Paper presented at the 60th Annual Scientific Conference of the Gerontological Society of America, 15–17 November, San Francisco.
Gorman-Murray, A. (2009) Intimate mobilities: emotional attachment and queer embodiment, *Social and Cultural Geography*, 10, 4, 441–60.
Grosz, E. (1994) *Volatile Bodies: towards a Corporeal Feminism*. Bloomington: Indiana University Press.
Hall, D. and Bytheway, B. (1982) The blocked bed: definition of a problem, *Social Science and Medicine*, 16, 1985–91.
Higgs, P. and Jones, I.R. (2008) *Medical Sociology and Old Age: towards a Sociology of Health in Later Life*. London: Routledge.
House of Commons (2007) Memorandum from the British Geriatrics Society, Ev 92; Oral Evidence, Ev 49–57, Ev 50, *The Human Rights of Older People in Healthcare*, Eighteenth Report of Session 2006–7, vol ll – Oral and Written Evidence, House of Lords and House of Commons Joint Committee on Human Rights, HL Paper 156-11, HC 378-ll.
Katz, S. (1996) *Disciplining Old Age: the Formation of Gerontological Knowledge*. Charlottesville: University Press of Virginia.
Martin, M. (1995) Medical knowledge and medical practice: geriatric medicine in the 1950s, *Social History of Medicine*, 8, 3, 443–61.
McVeigh, T. (2002) Scandal of NHS 'death factories', Guardian Unlimited. Available online at: http://www.guardian.co.uk/society/2002/aug/11/health.politics. Accessed 29.05.09.
Ministry of Health (1976) Recruitment to geriatric medicine, MH 149/1698, National Archives.
National Pensioners Convention (2009) Is the NHS caring for pensioners? *Campaign*, 29. Available online at: http://www.npcuk.org/campaigns/Campaign%20Bulletin%2029.pdf. Accessed 29.05.09
Phillipson, C. (2008) Authoring aging: Personal and social constructions, *Journal of Aging Studies*, 22, 163–68.
Phillipson, C. and Walker, A. (eds) (1998) *Ageing and Social Policy: a Critical Assessment*. Aldershot: Gower.
Phillipson, C. and Biggs, S. (1998) Modernity and identity: themes and perspectives in the study of older adults, *Journal of Aging and Identity*, 3, 1, 11–23.
Pitcher, B. (2008) The materiality of race theory, *Dark Matter*, available at: http://www.darkmatter101.org/site/2008/02/23/the-materiality-of-race-theory/ Accessed 5 June 2009

Puwar, N. (2004) *Space Invaders: Race, Gender, and Bodies out of Place*. Oxford: Berg.

Rivett, G. (1998) *From Cradle to Grave: Fifty Years of the NHS*. London: King's Fund.

Saldanha, A. (2006) Reontologising race: the machinic geography of phenotype, *Environment and Planning D: Society and Space*, 24, 9–24.

Skellington, D. (2008) Catalogue of disaster, *Guardian Unlimited*. Available online at: http://www.guardian.co.uk/society/2008/may/28/health.nhs. Accessed 29.05.09

Smith, D.J. (1980) *Overseas Doctors in the National Health Service*. London: Policy Studies Institute.

Thane, P. (2000) *Old Age in English History: Past Experiences, Present Issues*. Oxford: Oxford University Press.

Tulle, E. (2008) The ageing body and the ontology of ageing: athletic competence in later life, *Body and Society*, 14, 3, 1–19.

Turner, B (1984) *The Body and Society*, Blackwell, Oxford.

Turner, B. (1992) *Regulating Bodies: Essays in Medical Sociology*. New York: Routledge.

Twigg, J. (2000) *Bathing – the Body and Community Care*. London: Routledge.

Twigg, J. (2002) The body in social policy: mapping a territory, *Journal of Social Policy*, 31, 3, 421–39.

Twigg, J. (2004) The body, gender and age: feminist insights in social gerontology, *Journal of Aging Studies*, 18, 59–73.

Veninga, C. (2009) Fitting in: the embodied politics of race in Seattle's desegregated schools, *Social and Cultural Geography*, 10, 2, 107–29.

Vincent, J. (2007) Science and imagery in the 'war on old age', *Ageing and Society*, 27, 6, 941–61.

Vincent, J. (2008) The cultural construction of old age as a biological phenomenon: science and anti-ageing technologies, *Journal of Aging Studies*, 22, 331–9.

Warren, M. (1943) Care of chronic sick: a case for treating chronic sick in blocks in a general hospital, *British Medical Journal*, 2, ii, 822–3.

Wolkowitz, C. (2006) *Bodies at Work*. London: Sage.

Yancy, G. (2008) Elevators, social spaces and racism: a philosophical analysis, *Philosophy and Social Criticism*, 34, 843–76.

12

Afterword: Body work and the sociological tradition
Chris Shilling

Introduction

Body Work in Health and Social Care: Critical Themes, New Agendas is a welcome addition to the social scientific literature in the field of 'body studies', demonstrating as it does the importance of the body to one of the longest standing areas of sociological interest, work. By focusing on the inter-corporeal tensions, challenges, co-operations, pleasures, ambivalences and emotional exchanges associated with *bodies-working-on-bodies*, the chapters in this volume combine original empirical research with a theoretical sensitivity towards social, cultural and phenomenological issues relevant to our understanding of this type of labour. Such an accomplishment is particularly timely as the importance of body work to the economy appears to have grown alongside the expansion of the service sector. Depending on the definition of 'body work' or 'interactive body work' utilised, it is estimated that between 10 per cent and 30 per cent of all jobs in Britain alone now involve this type of activity (Wolkowitz 2006, Cohen 2008, McDowell 2009). Ranging from the caring and welfare services, to the commercialisation of domestic labour and the expansion of sex work, to the large growth in cosmetic surgery/procedures that has taken place over the last decade, body work is significant for the formal economy and the hidden economy.

In this context, the issues raised within *Body Work in Health and Social Care* are not just of academic concern, but deserve the attention of politicians and policy makers, front-line workers, and recipients of health, welfare and other body-related services. This judgment is justified by the briefest summary of several key problems covered by the contributors to this volume; problems that include the stratification of the body work sector in terms of its prestige and stigma (Raghuram *et al.*), the corporeal conditions delimiting the temporal, spatial and rational organisation of body work (Cohen, and England and Dyck), and the 'interaction order' of body work (Brown *et al.*). By exploring such subjects, this volume also analyses the difficulties of achieving control of one's own and other people's bodies during therapy/treatment (Cacchioni and Wolkowitz, Tarr, and Gale), how alterations in technology can block the effective deployment of habits that previously facilitated the effective operation of body-machine assemblages (Harris, and Måseide), and the processes involved in learning physical techniques capable of achieving effective working linkages with other body subjects (Wainwright).

Body Work in Health and Social Care, First Edition. Edited by Julia Twigg, Carol Wolkowitz, Rachel Lara Cohen and Sarah Nettleton.

These studies have a refreshingly contemporary feel to them, and it is easy to view the area of body work in general as possessing only recent origins (Shilling 1993: 118). To do so would be a mistake, though, as the analyses within *Body Work in Health and Social Care* possess affinities with a wealth of classical explorations into the relationship between economic, social and cultural activity, on the one hand, and the broader contexts in which work occurs involving the shaping, socialising, training, treating, exciting, caring, maintaining and decorating of bodies, on the other. While current interest in contemporary forms of body work has added important insights to sociology and social policy, then, it is important that this research is not undertaken in the context of an amnesia regarding what has already been accomplished. Classical sociological contributions to body work may demand a wider definition of the subject than that employed in this volume, but they reinforce the social and cultural significance of bodies-working-on-bodies, illustrate the centrality of this phenomenon to the core concerns of the discipline, and highlight broader issues with which current studies on body work might engage. In the remainder of this brief Afterword, I want simply to illustrate these points by suggesting that the shaping and steering of the health, habits, emotions and other characteristics of individuals that occurs during body work is integrally related to issues that have been central to the sociological tradition.

Body work in sociology

Of most immediate relevance in assessing the significance of body work, perhaps, is the central theme that runs through Marx's *Economic and Philosophical Manuscripts of 1844*, is developed in *The German Ideology*, and is explored empirically in the context of industrialisation within Engels's *The Condition of the Working Class in England*: embodied subjects produce *themselves* and *others* through their *labour*. Marx (1954: 173) explored how this 'setting in motion' of our 'arms and legs, heads and hands' could benefit the corporeal capacities and dispositions of ourselves and others, yet was most focused upon explicating how capitalist relations and forces of production damaged and alienated individuals from the creative potential of their own, and other people's, physical being, and turned body subjects into the appendages of machines (Marx 1975: 329–30, 1968: 41).

If Marx was the first figure now recognised widely as core to sociology to state the general importance of the mutually transformative relationship that exists between work and embodied subjects, it is also worth reminding ourselves of Durkheim's specific concern with the role of the body in the reproduction of societies, and Weber's explorations of the development of a *habitus* suited to rational capitalism. Both accounts highlight the importance of body work for central sociological issues.

Durkheim is renowned for his analyses of how societies are reproduced through collective assemblies, phases of social life that reinforce the idea and feeling of *belonging* to a moral order, but the significance of body work to this process is still being explicated (Shilling and Mellor 2011). Collective assemblies involve people congregating together in the presence of totemic representations of what they consider to be sacred; representations that stimulate intense, effervescent emotions, and assume their 'most important' form when *imprinted on* and *assimilated into* the flesh of participants (Durkheim 1995: 114, 218–22). The ritualised, inter-corporeal marking and socialising of body subjects that occur during these assemblies steer the emotional effervescence they provoke, and ensure that participants come to imagine and experience 'the society of which they are a part' (Durkheim 1995: 229). Collective life, in short, is reproduced through participants' *bodies*; bodies that have been *worked upon* by, and are also intoxicated by, the ritual bodily actions of others (Shilling 2005).

Developed through an engagement with ethnographic materials on Aboriginal totemism, Durkheim's theory has been applied to contemporary nationalistic, sporting and other ceremonies (*e.g.* Mestrovic 1993), but it is Weber's (1991) analysis of the body work associated with the Protestant Ethic that provides us with the most productive theoretical account of how an *early modern* habitus came to be fitted for work within rational capitalism. Motivated by a search for signs of election in the fruits of their labour, and a religious ethos equating sensuality with sin, Protestantism sought to reform habits through an ascetic disciplining of body subjects: long hours of labour were validated as means of living righteously, diary keeping was promoted as a means of monitoring thoughts and actions, and regulations and laws were directed towards the control of personal life. As Weber (1991: 36) argues, the reformers sought to regulate 'the whole of conduct which penetrated to all depths of private and public life'. This Protestant attempt to promote disciplined body subjects was uneven (Roper 1994), but it does not diminish the importance of the gradual internalisation of new codes of behaviour and orientations to the body that occured in the early modern era (Mellor and Shilling 1997).

The contributions of classical writers such as Marx, Durkheim and Weber emanate from contrasting philosophical traditions, and are predicated upon opposing methodological assumptions. While their contributions remain generally focused upon the broad contexts in which body work occurs, they provide us with indications of its longstanding sociological importance. For those concerned with more finely grained analyses of how the economy, society and culture get translated into, and relate to, specific forms of body work, however, it is worth looking to other sources of sociological inspiration.

Body techniques, body pedagogics
Irrespective of their differences, Marx, Durkheim and Weber were interested in how bodies are 'worked upon' – in part by other body subjects – in varying social contexts; contexts that relate to the development of capitalist production, the constitution of collectivities, and the economic consequences of socio-religious movements. It is Marcel Mauss, though, who has was one of the most astute commentators on those specific processes whereby the external environments of human action get translated into the activities, postures, tensions, appearances and actions of embodied subjects.

Viewing the body as the individual's first and most natural object, and techniques as actions that are 'effective' within a particular inter-corporeal and natural environment, Mauss (1973: 70) employs the term 'techniques of the body' to identify '[t]he way in which from society to society' people 'know how to use their bodies'. Bodily techniques of working, walking, conversing, swimming, caring, nurturing, praying and even breathing are not natural or universal, but vary historically and cross-culturally. They involve social, biological and psychological components, and are acquired initially through a process of 'prestigious imitation' in which the child or adult copies 'actions which have succeeded and which he has seen successfully performed by people in whom he has confidence and who have authority over him' (Mauss 1973: 73). This imitation is complemented and reinforced, however, by the physical encouragement, instruction, steering and guidance that occurs during body work, translating imitation into incorporation (*e.g.* Lande 2007). The body work that occurs during infant socialisation, and the inculcation of young adults into working life, for example, involves physical corrections and discipline that constitute an 'education in composure', a means of assisting the control of emotions, and a way of allowing 'a co-ordinated response of co-ordinated movements setting off in the direction of a chosen goal' (Mauss 1973: 86, see also Elias 2000).

Mauss's (1973) analysis of the techniques employed within forms of body work characteristic of a society is relevant to those questions of economics, culture and religion explored by the founding figures. Furthermore, despite his Durkheimian roots, Mauss's concern with how body techniques are manifest in *individual* body subjects, mediated by *social interaction*, and informed not only by social *norms* but by the technical efficiency with which they enable people to intervene in the world, makes his work relevant to a range of sociological methodologies. In terms of our concern with body work, then, Mauss allows us to understand how the manner in which individuals work on the bodies of others is not just of interpersonal significance. Instead, through the impact it has on the formation of behavioural habits and the habitus of embodied subjects, he demonstrates how body work also has implications for major structural issues within sociology and social policy. What Mauss argues is that body work involves an education, or a *pedagogics*, that directs people's activities along certain pathways, and away from others, establishing certain actions as habits while blocking the routinisation of others (Shilling and Mellor 2007). It is these physical habits that are key not only to the micro-processes involved in body work, but to the future of society, culture and the economy.

In conclusion, it is worth noting that Mauss's engagement with habits highlights a key theme within *Body Work in Health and Social Care*. Habits are modes of connection, unifying us with other people in particular ways and, in the case of body work, shaping people's embodied health, appearance, pleasures, pains and capacities in particular directions. Far from being neutral in relation to the broader issues central to the writings of Marx, Weber, Durkheim and other classical sociologists, they involve a 'special sensitiveness' to 'certain classes of stimuli', demanding 'certain kinds of activity', and steering our behaviour towards certain types of social, cultural and economic organisation, while also closing off other possibilities (James 1950: 114, Dewey 2002 [1922]: 125).

If the construction of habits through the work of bodies on bodies is a key contribution of *Body Work in Health and Social Care*, its analyses also usefully demonstrate the difficulties of acquiring these habits, and the obstacles individuals can confront in exercising them. Habits clash, and can become ineffective, and ossify as bodies age and decay, and as the technologies and the environments with which they connect change. Embodied action, and body work, is not confined to the deployment and inculcation of habits, but cycles through periods and stages of crisis and creativity in response to various factors (Shilling 2008). These changes are not just consequential for the individuals concerned, but have major implications for those issues raised by Marx, Weber, Durkheim and others whose writings enable us to connect through the subject of body work the minutae of individual action with the 'structural' issues of society, culture and the economy.

References

Cohen, R.L. (2008) Body work, employment relations and the labour process, paper presented at ESRC Seminar *Body Work*. University of Warwick, 18–19 January.
Dewey, J. (2002 [1922]) *Human Nature and Conduct*. New York: Dover.
McDowell, L. (2009) *Working Bodies*. Oxford: Wiley-Blackwell.
James, W. (1950 [1890]) *The Principles of Psychology*. Two Volumes. New York: Dover.
Durkheim, E. (1995) *The Elementary Forms of Religious Life*. New York: Free Press.

Elias, N. (2000 [1939]) *The Civilizing Process*. Oxford: Blackwell.
Lande, B. (2007) Breathing like a soldier: culture incarnate. In Shilling, C. (ed.) *Embodying Sociology*. Oxford: Blackwell.
Marx, K. (1954 [1867]) *Capital*, Volume 1. London: Lawrence and Wisharrt.
Marx, K. (1975 [1844]) The economic and philosophic manuscripts of 1844. In Marx, K. (ed.) *Early Writings*. London: Penguin.
Mauss, M. (1973 [1934]) Techniques of the body, *Economy and Society* 2, 70–88.
Mellor, P.A. and Shilling, C. (1997) *Re-forming the Body. Religion Community and Modernity*. London: Sage.
Mestrovic, S. (1993) *The Barbarian Temperament*. London: Routledge.
Roper, L. (1994) *Oedipus and the Devil*. London: Routledge.
Shilling, C. (1993) *The Body and Social Theory*. London: Sage.
Shilling, C. (2005) Embodiment, emotions and the foundations of social order: Durkheim's enduring contribution. In Alexander, J. and Smith, P. (eds) *The Cambridge Companion to Emile Durkheim*. Cambridge: Cambridge University Press.
Shilling, C. (2008) *Changing Bodies. Habit, Crisis and Creativity*. London: Sage.
Shilling, C. and Mellor, P.A. (2007) Cultures of embodied experience: technology, religion and body pedagogics, *The Sociological Review*, 55, 3, 531–49.
Shilling, C. and Mellor, P.A. (2011) Embodiment, intoxication and collective life: Emile Durkheim on society and religion, *The Sociological Review*. Forthcoming.
Weber, M. (1991 [1904–05]) *The Protestant Ethic and the Spirit of Capitalism*. London: Macmillan.
Wolkowitz, C. (2006) *Body Work*. London: Routledge.

Index

Note: page numbers in *italics* denote a figure/table.

Body Work in Health and Social Care, First Edition. Edited by Julia Twigg, Carol Wolkowitz, Rachel Lara Cohen and Sarah Nettleton.
Chapters © 2011 The Authors. Book compilation © 2011 Foundation for the Sociology of Health & Illness / Blackwell Publishing Ltd. Published 2011 by Blackwell Publishing Ltd.